Jean Betschart Roemer, MN, MSN, CRNP, CDE

AMERICAN DIABETES ASSOCIATION

Guide to Raising a Child with Diabetes

THIRD EDITION

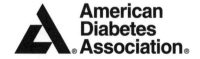

Director/Book Publishing; Abe Ogden; *Acquisitions Editor,* Victor Van Beuren; *Editor,* Rebekah Renshaw; *Production Manager,* Melissa Sprott; *Composition,* ADA; *Cover Design,* Pixiedesign, Inc.; *Printer,* United Graphics.

Printed in the United States of America
1 3 5 7 9 10 8 6 4 2

The suggestions and information contained in this publication are generally consistent with the *Clinical Practice Recommendations* and other policies of the American Diabetes Association, but they do not represent the policy or position of the Association or any of its boards or committees. Reasonable steps have been taken to ensure the accuracy of the information presented. However, the American Diabetes Association cannot ensure the safety or efficacy of any product or service described in this publication. Individuals are advised to consult a physician or other appropriate health care professional before undertaking any diet or exercise program or taking any medication referred to in this publication. Professionals must use and apply their own professional judgment, experience, and training and should not rely solely on the information contained in this publication before prescribing any diet, exercise, or medication. The American Diabetes Association—its officers, directors, employees, volunteers, and members—assumes no responsibility or liability for personal or other injury, loss, or damage that may result from the suggestions or information in this publication.

♾ The paper in this publication meets the requirements of the ANSI Standard Z39.48-1992 (permanence of paper).

ADA titles may be purchased for business or promotional use or for special sales. To purchase more than 50 copies of this book at a discount, or for custom editions of this book with your logo, contact the American Diabetes Association at the address below, at booksales@diabetes.org, or by calling 703-299-2046.

American Diabetes Association
1701 North Beauregard Street
Alexandria, Virginia 22311

Library of Congress Cataloging-in-Publication Data
Betschart-Roemer, Jean, 1948-
  American Diabetes Association guide to raising a child with diabetes / Jean Betschart Roemer.—3rd ed.
    p. cm.
  Summary: "This book is written to provide the reader with reassurance and sound informa-tion so that they can make wise decisions in the daily life and care of a child with diabetes. It contains information for parents of children and others caring for a child with type 1 diabetes, although many of the developmental issues and treatments can also apply to the ever-growing population of type 2 diabetes in youth"-- Provided by publisher.
  Rev. ed. of: American Diabetes Association guide to raising a child with diabetes / Linda Siminerio, Jean Betschart. 2nd ed.
  Includes bibliographical references and index.
  ISBN 978-1-58040-435-8 (pbk.)
  1. Diabetes in children--Popular works. 2. Diabetes in children--Patients--Home care. I. Siminerio, Linda M. American Diabetes Association guide to raising a child with diabetes. II. Title. III. Title: Guide to raising a child with diabetes.
  RJ420.D5S57 2011
  618.92'462--dc22
                          2010041425

Dedication

To Linda M. Siminerio, PhD, my friend and colleague, who co-authored earlier editions, and her father, John A. Mulac, to whom she dedicated those editions; and to the loving memory of my daughter, Julie Betschart (1972–1997), in honor of my daughter Kelly Vokoun, MD, and son, Jeff Betschart, BA, RN.

Acknowledgments

Thanks to the following people for reviewing this edition of *Guide to Raising a Child with Diabetes:* Kathy Cashin, MSN, RN, CDE; Janis Roszler, RD, CDE, LD/N; and Joan Hill, RD, CDE, LD.

I extend special thanks to my husband for his support of my writings and projects to promote diabetes care, to the members of the Children's Hospital of Pittsburgh Diabetes Care Team for their encouragement, to God for giving me the ability, and to the American Diabetes Association for their pursuit of excellence.

Thanks to Rebekah Renshaw for her expertise and great editing suggestions. Thanks also to Victor Van Beuren for giving me the encouragement and opportunity to write this edition.

Table of Contents

Preface

Raising a child in today's world is a challenge all by itself. Our fast-paced lives leave little room to deal with normal childhood issues, let alone complex ones. If your child develops diabetes, adding the concerns of diabetes care to all of the other tasks, obligations, and joys of parenting might cause you to feel overwhelmed.

My purpose in writing this book is to provide you with reassurance and information so you can make wise decisions in the daily life and care of your child with diabetes. This book is for parents or those caring for a child with type 1 diabetes, although many of the developmental issues and treatments can also apply to the ever-growing population of type 2 diabetes in youth. A section on type 2 diabetes is included in this book (see page 127) and addresses the differences and special needs of the child with type 2 diabetes.

I hope that you find the information and tools to deal with everyday situations as they arise, along with an understanding about how your child's age and development impact diabetes management. My goal is for you to become confident about your ability to raise a child with diabetes.

The best diabetes care is somewhat structured, yet flexible and dynamic. Ideally, you will be able to fit diabetes care into the routines of everyday life, and yet modify it as your child grows and develops. Food preferences come and go. Children pick up different hobbies and sports. Your approach to diabetes care will need to change based on the needs of your child, the philosophy of your health care team, and your own parenting style. Help can come from many sources: loving friends and relatives; a strong, caring medical team; and the knowledge you gather as you learn as much as you possibly can about diabetes. As your child grows and changes, the way diabetes affects her life will change as well.

Use the guidance here in conjunction with the advice of your health care providers. These are guidelines based on what experience and research have shown to be effective. Since insulin was first discovered, education has been a cornerstone of diabetes treatment. The more you and your child know about diabetes and how to treat it, the better equipped you will be to make wise decisions.

There are many successful ways to treat diabetes. If you are currently doing something different from what is recommended here, it does not mean that one way is right or the other wrong. The right approach is the one that works best for your child and your family. Sometimes, the only way of knowing which approach is best is to try several different strategies.

I have alternated the use of he and she by chapters to avoid having to repeat the awkward "he or she" when referring to your child. Also, any mention of a brand name product does not imply endorsement of the product by the American Diabetes Association or myself. Brand names, when used, are only examples of the types of products available.

Jean Betschart Roemer

Introduction

R esearch is moving forward to find a cure. Even though there is no cure for diabetes at this time, continuing advancements are making control easier. New and better kinds of insulin are available. Easy-to-use glucose meters make it possible for children to check their own blood glucose levels quickly and easily with very small amounts of blood. Syringes are more comfortable than ever; state-of-the-art insulin pumps and continuous glucose sensors are now available. The list goes on as technological advances are exploding! New knowledge gained from research tells us that diabetes treatment can be flexible, that rigid diets and schedules are not always necessary, and that diligence pays off in the treatment of diabetes and the prevention of future health problems.

Diabetes should not keep your child from achieving her highest goals. There are Olympic athletes, professional football players, members of congress, actors, and rock stars who live with diabetes Some examples are: Jay Cutler (NFL quarterback), Nick Jonas (Jonas Brothers), Joe Gibbs (former NFL coach), Halle Berry (actress), and Anne Rice (author). The good news is that you and your child can successfully adjust to life with diabetes. Diabetes affects many, but doesn't have to slow your child down or limit what they can do. Encourage your children to follow their dreams.

When you learn that your child has diabetes, you might think that life has turned upside down. There is too much information to absorb when you are in emotional shock, and you don't know enough to ask the right questions. You need to grasp the basic concepts of high and low blood glucose, learn to give an injection to your child, and monitor and treat his low blood glucose levels. Parents report this period of time as being very stressful, especially when the diagnosis comes without warning.

Parents often feel some responsibility and even some guilt over their child's development of diabetes. We tend to believe that "good" parenting means protecting your child from harm; keeping her safe. These efforts are intended to control the environment and prevent anything harmful from happening to our children. So when a child develops a chronic illness, you, as the provider and protector, probably feel as though you should have or could have done something to prevent it. You might feel helpless in the face of your child's illness.

Accept that there was nothing you could have done to prevent the onset of your child's type 1 diabetes. You will need to find a firm footing, dig in, and make the best of things without feeling guilty. Even if you had known that your child was genetically at risk for diabetes, currently, there is no known way of preventing the disease from occurring.

Allow yourself time to be sad about the diagnosis. The disease will impact your life and the life of your child in many ways, and although it is treatable and you should have every reason to be optimistic about your child's future, it is still a loss that needs to be grieved. Keep in mind that diabetes is manageable and it doesn't have to keep you and your child from living life to the fullest.

As you live with diabetes, you may also feel guilt about not keeping to a schedule, allowing your child to eat foods that are not the healthiest, being too firm about not allowing certain foods, and the pricks and finger sticks of daily management. Although these feelings are normal, allow yourself the luxury of the question, "Am I doing the best that I can under the circumstances?" If the answer is "yes," try not to obsess over it, and move on. When you have a family, it is difficult to focus on one family member when there are others who also demand time and attention. Be forgiving of yourself, call out your support team (or create one), and deal with it the best you can.

Controlling diabetes can indeed be a challenge, because blood glucose levels can vary in spite of your best efforts. You can do everything right, follow all the instructions from your doctor, educator, and dietitian, and your child's blood glucose may still not be where you want it to be. On the other hand, things may go well when you least expect them to. This is frustrating and puzzling. Keeping records, trying different approaches, being a good problem-solver, and maintaining some consistency of schedule and daily life can be helpful to understanding patterns. Learning as much as you can and keeping records will help you to make good decisions.

CHAPTER 1:
What Is Diabetes?

Chapter 1:
What Is Diabetes?

Diabetes mellitus is not a new disease. It was around as early as 30 A.D. Diabetes is a Greek word that means "to run through." Mellitus is a Latin word that means "honeyed." Healers coined this term to describe what they saw: people with diabetes urinated a lot and their urine was sweet. Before the discovery of insulin in1922, children might live up to a year after diagnosis of diabetes and died of starvation or dehydration. At that time, people thought insulin was "the cure," but we now know that not to be the case. Insulin is the treatment, and researchers are still working hard to find the cure. Despite recent progress in our understanding of the genetics and immune process of the disease, diabetes continues to increase by a rate of 3–5% per year.

Diabetes occurs when the body cannot use and store food properly due to a lack of insulin or inability to use the insulin being made. Insulin is a hormone made in the beta cells of the pancreas. It allows the body to use glucose for energy. Food is made up of protein, carbohydrate, and fats. When food is digested, it is broken down so that

> "Diabetes continues to increase by a rate of 3–5% per year."

Diabetes in Children

Diabetes is one of the most common chronic diseases in children. Type 1 diabetes is the third most common chronic disease of childhood after asthma and cystic fibrosis. In the United States, there are approximately 216,000 children and teens under the age of 20 who have diabetes (type 1 or type 2). This represents 0.26% of all people in this age group. Estimates of undiagnosed diabetes are unavailable for this age group.

it can be used for energy. Proteins are broken down into amino acids. Carbohydrates become glucose. Fats become fatty acids. All of these particles enter your bloodstream and travel through the body to feed cells.

Glucose is the body's main energy source, made from both carbohydrates and proteins. Before it can be used as energy, glucose must move inside the body's cells. Insulin is the key that allows glucose to move through the cell wall and enter the cell.

In people with diabetes, either the body does not make enough, or any, insulin, or it cannot use the insulin available. In type 1 diabetes, the beta cells in the pancreas are destroyed and no longer produce insulin. So, instead of entering the cells, glucose stays in the blood. The cells starve, and glucose levels in the blood rise. A high glucose level in the blood (also known as hyperglycemia) is a sign of diabetes.

The two most common types of diabetes are type 1 and type 2 diabetes. In type 1 diabetes, the body doesn't make enough (or any) insulin. People with this type of diabetes depend on daily injections of insulin to survive. It is diagnosed more often in children and teens but can be diagnosed well into adulthood. The onset of type 1 appears to be rapid; however, scientists have found that the development is a multi-year process. People who develop type 1 are born with a genetic risk of developing it.

In type 2 diabetes, the body makes insulin but doesn't use it properly. Being overweight and inactive are risk factors in people who are genetically susceptible. The causes of type 2 diabetes are a combination of heredity, ethnic origin, excess weight, sedentary lifestyle, history of gestational diabetes, and giving birth to a baby over 9 pounds.

Insulin resistance develops over time, leading to an inability to maintain normal blood glucose level. Many of the signs of high blood glucose are the same in both type 1 and type 2 diabetes. People with type 2 diabetes can often manage their diabetes by watching the quantity and type of food they eat, increasing exercise, and taking an oral medication. Often, they also need to take medications such as insulin.

Because children, teens, and adults in the United States and many other countries around the globe are fighting excess weight, in recent years, there has been a tremendous upsurge in the number of children and teens diagnosed with type 2 diabetes.

THE PANCREAS

To understand type 1 diabetes you need to know about the pancreas, a large gland located behind the stomach. The pancreas has two main jobs. It makes digestive juices and chemicals called enzymes that break down food for use as fuel. The pancreas also makes hormones that help to deliver fuel to cells. One of these hormones is insulin, which delivers glucose to cells.

Clusters of cells in the pancreas are called the islets of Langerhans. The islets are made up of beta cells, which make insulin. Type 1 diabetes occurs when the beta cells are destroyed and can no longer make insulin. This process can be gradual or abrupt. Without insulin, the body cannot use glucose for energy. Insulin by injection or insulin pump replaces the missing insulin and allows the body to use glucose.

CAUSES OF TYPE 1 DIABETES

Type 1 diabetes is an autoimmune disease. An autoimmune illness is one where the body rejects and destroys its own cells, almost like having an allergy to yourself. The reasons why the beta cells stop making insulin are not well understood; however, it is known that the destruction is due to an autoimmune process. This means that antibodies are produced that destroy the beta cells that make insulin.

Other types of autoimmune diseases include: lupus, thyroid disease, multiple sclerosis, celiac disease, vitiligo (skin disease), and even a form of baldness. In these diseases, the body produces antibodies in response to a viral or environmental trigger and these antibodies mistakenly attack and injure a part of the body. In the case of type 1 diabetes, the antibodies attack the insulin-making cells in the pancreas, and eventually destroy them so that insulin is no longer made. These antibodies can be present for long periods of time before signs of diabetes appear. Scientists don't know exactly how a virus might lead to diabetes; however, they do know that some people inherit a higher risk for type 1 diabetes. Some families have more than one member with diabetes because family members share the genes that make them prone to diabetes.

Current studies are looking at families to see if other family members have the antibodies and whether we can predict with greater certainty those who may go on to develop diabetes. Diabetes is also related to certain inherited genes. Genetic typing (DNA sequencing) suggests a high or low risk of developing type 1 diabetes. Genes alone do not seem to cause type 1 diabetes, but they do determine your risk of developing diabetes. It's possible that in people whose genes make them prone to diabetes, a virus or other stressor causes the antibody destruction that leads to diabetes.

> "Some people, especially children, worry that they can 'catch' diabetes. Diabetes is not contagious."

Other studies are investigating what starts the process in the first place, what can be done to protect the cells that make insulin, and why some people can have antibodies yet not have clinical signs of diabetes. Some people, especially children, worry that they can "catch" diabetes from contact with someone who has it. Diabetes is not contagious. It cannot be transmitted from one person to another.

Many children who get diabetes do so shortly after having a viral illness. The peak months for the diagnosis of diabetes in children are September, January, and February, paralleling cold and flu season. The virus may have caused the autoimmune response, or the children may have been going to get diabetes anyway, and the viral illness brought it on quickly. Thousands of children get viral infections every year, and only a few of them get diabetes.

SIGNS AND SYMPTOMS OF DIABETES

The symptoms of diabetes are caused by blood glucose levels that are too high (hyperglycemia). When the body stops making insulin and high blood glucose is not treated with insulin, a condition called ketoacidosis may develop. Ketoacidosis is a very serious condition and must be treated quickly by doctors and nurses experienced with diabetes in children. The symptoms associated with high blood glucose levels (see page 8) or ketoacidosis are often the first indication of diabetes. Experiencing these symptoms may be what brought you and your child to the doctor or hospital when your child was first diagnosed.

Hyperglycemia (High Blood Glucose)

Hyperglycemia is a high level of glucose in the blood and is a sign of uncontrolled diabetes. Here's what happens: after food is eaten, the digestive process breaks it down into glucose. Normally, insulin helps to move glucose from the blood into the body's cells. Insulin is like the doorman that opens the cell doors, letting the glucose in. People with type 1 diabetes don't make insulin, so glucose stays in their blood instead of entering the cells. People with type 2 diabetes often have a lot of insulin, but it is unable to enter the cells, so it cannot travel inside the cells and will remain in their blood. The cells then begin to starve and glucose builds up in the blood. Blood glucose levels can go too high when your child:

♦ gets too little insulin, too much food, or too little exercise
♦ is under physical stress from a cold, sore throat, or other illness
♦ is feeling emotional stress.

The human body is always working toward a state of balance. When there is an emergency state in one system, other systems go into action to help. When the cells are starving, this is an emergency state. Untreated, hyperglycemia can lead to ketoacidosis. It's important to work with your health care provider to develop a plan to get and keep your blood glucose levels under control. When your child develops diabetes, she may have some or all of the signs (see Symptoms of Hyperglycemia, next page) that indicate her blood glucose level is too high. You will learn to recognize the signs and symptoms of hyperglycemia in your child. (For information on how to prevent and treat hyperglycemia, see page 115.)

Ketoacidosis and Diabetic Coma

As the signs and symptoms of high blood glucose progress and worsen, the body literally begins to starve. Your child can slip into a state known as diabetic ketoacidosis or "DKA." This serious condition is an emergency and demands rapid treatment. Without insulin, glucose cannot enter the body's cells to provide energy. The cells are forced to burn fat to get the energy they need. When fat is burned, by-products called ketones build up in the blood and spill into the urine.

Symptoms of Hyperglycemia

♦ Frequent urination. When your child has diabetes, high glucose in the blood spills into the urine, pulling water with it. This creates a large volume of urine and makes your child urinate a lot. You may not be aware of it during the day, but increased urination at night and bedwetting is often what captures a parent's attention.

♦ Excessive thirst. As sugar and water are pulled into the urine, dehydration begins and thirst develops. You may notice that your child becomes extremely thirsty, drinking glass upon glass of liquids. If he is drinking sweetened liquids, it makes him even more thirsty.

♦ Increased appetite. This is the body's way of asking for the food it needs to maintain weight and replace calories lost in urine.

♦ Weight loss. Your child may lose weight because the body, unable to make proper use of food, tries to get nourishment by burning stored fat for energy. Weight loss also occurs due to dehydration because the body is losing so much water in urine.

♦ Tiredness and weakness. Your child may feel tired and weak because the body's cells are dehydrated and starving. Muscle cramping may occur. Muscles and other tissues are depleted of glucose and water.

♦ Vision problems. Your child may complain of difficulty seeing the chalkboard or reading signs at a distance. High blood glucose can cause the lens of the eye to change shape, leading to blurred vision. This does not cause permanent eye damage and is not an eye complication. Once her blood glucose is under control, your child's vision should return to normal.

Small amounts of ketones are probably not harmful; however, when ketones build up they cause the blood to turn acidic, which can act like poison. A high level of ketones in the blood and urine is called ketoacidosis. The most common causes of ketoacidosis are:

♦ undiagnosed or newly diagnosed diabetes

♦ illness

♦ too little insulin to meet the body's needs

If left untreated, ketoacidosis can lead to a coma, brain swelling, and even death. With prompt treatment, children usually recover from ketoacidosis without any after effects at all. (For more on preventing and treating ketoacidosis, see page 116.) If your child did not have these signs and symptoms when she was initially diagnosed, the most likely time to see them would be during an illness, or if insulin has been omitted. Your child will appear quite ill as symptoms worsen and will need emergency care.

Warning Signs of Ketoacidosis

Ketoacidosis usually does not develop without warning. The signs and symptoms of ketoacidosis are:

♦ ketones in the urine and blood

♦ dehydration (symptoms include sunken eyes; dry, cracked lips; dry mouth; and skin that remains pinched up after it is pinched)

♦ nausea and vomiting

♦ fruity-smelling breath

♦ rapid or heavy breathing

♦ abdominal pain

♦ extreme drowsiness

If your child develops any of these symptoms, it's extremely important to contact your doctor right away.

Hypoglycemia (Low Blood Glucose)

Hypoglycemia, or low blood glucose levels, can occur once treatment for diabetes has begun. Hypoglycemia must be treated quickly with carbohydrate to raise blood glucose to a normal range. Low blood glucose occurs when your child's insulin dose is too large, he hasn't eaten enough food (or has eaten late), or he has exercised more than usual.

When blood glucose starts to drop too low, adrenaline (a hormone that helps the body deal with emergencies) jumps into action to try to raise it. When this happens, your child may show some of the following signs and symptoms, which are related to this rush of adrenaline:

- pale, clammy skin
- sweating
- rapid pulse
- shakiness
- tingling
- hunger

Many young children do not recognize or report symptoms when they occur. This unawareness puts them at greater risk for having more severe hypoglycemia. Just as you will learn to recognize the symptoms of high blood glucose in your child, you will also learn to recognize the symptoms of low blood glucose. (For how to prevent and treat hypoglycemia, see page 105.) By talking to your young child about how he felt (hungry, tired, shaky, etc) you will help him learn to recognize symptoms.

KEEP BLOOD GLUCOSE IN A TARGET RANGE

For a person without diabetes, a normal blood glucose range is between 70–99 mg/dl. While a normal target range for adults with diabetes is between 70–130 mg/dl, the acceptable ranges are typically higher for children and some adolescents because of the unique risks of hypoglycemia unawareness in young children. A laboratory blood test called A1C shows a person's average blood glucose level over the past 60

Symptoms of Severe Hypoglycemia

Most of the time hypoglycemia is mild and can be easily treated by giving your child something containing sugar to eat or drink (see list of foods for treating hypoglycemia, page 113). In severe hypoglycemia, the brain is deprived of glucose, causing the following symptoms:

- headache
- personality changes
- irritability, crying
- poor coordination
- seizures/unconsciousness

- confusion
- nightmares
- fatigue, sleepiness
- dizziness

days. Normal, non-diabetic levels are usually below 6.1%. (See page 12 for A1C guidelines for your child's age.)

Although we now know that keeping blood glucose levels close to normal helps to prevent the complications of diabetes, it is very difficult to always maintain a normal level when insulin is given rather than made within one's own pancreas. It is difficult if not impossible to keep all values within the normal range in a child with type 1 diabetes. The goal is to keep blood glucose as low as possible without frequent or severe low blood glucose.

Decide what your child's blood glucose target should be with your health care provider. If your child/teen is old enough, he should participate in the decision. You should all come to an agreement on what is reasonable for your child and figure out the target range you will shoot for. Some parents are extremely fearful of low blood glucose because of a past experience, so it is important to tell your doctor about your concerns. A host of factors can impact blood glucose numbers, such as how quickly insulin is absorbed from different body sites, how quickly food is digested and used, the type of foods eaten, the type of activity or exercise, stress, and many more factors.

Goals for Type 1 Diabetes by Age Group (A1C and Blood Glucose)

| Values By Age (years) | Blood Glucose Goal Range | | A1C | Rationale |
	Before meals	Bedtime/overnight		
Toddlers and preschoolers (0–6)	100–180	110–200	<8.5% (but >7.5%)	–High risk and vulnerability to hypoglycemia
School age (6–12)	90–180	100–180	<8%	–Risks of hypoglycemia and relatively low risk of complications prior to puberty
Adolescents and young adults (13–19)	90–130	90–150	<7.5%	–Risk of severe hypoglycemia –Development and psychological issues –A lower goal (<7.0%) is reasonable if achieved without excessive hypoglycemia

Key concepts in setting glycemic goals:

◆ Goals should be individualized and lower goals may be reasonable based on benefit–risk assessment.

◆ Blood glucose goals should be higher than those listed above in children with frequent hypoglycemia.

(Adapted from American Diabetes Association Clinical Practice Recommendations, 2010.)

There are times when your child's blood glucose will be well within the range, and other times when it's outside the range. Sometimes you will know why your child's blood glucose was out of range and other times you won't. Try to determine if there is a reason behind the high or low blood glucose, but know that there isn't always a reason. If you can't figure it out, it's okay. Sometimes blood glucose bounces and no one knows exactly why, especially in children.

You and your child will have days where your blood glucose numbers are terrific, along with challenging days. You will get frustrated at times. Diabetes can be unpredictable. Sometimes things may not go well even when you do everything right. On the other hand, glucose levels may stay in range when you don't expect them to, such as on a day when your child has a party or her usual schedule is disrupted. The reasons for high and low blood sugar levels are not always apparent because there are too many possible reasons or causes in everyday life that cannot be controlled. How insulin is absorbed, the type and quantity of carbohydrate eaten, amount of protein, fat, and fiber eaten, differences in types of sports and exercise, and hormonal effects due to stress and puberty all impact blood glucose levels.

A problem-solving approach to diabetes management is important for you and your child. If you can figure out what caused the unusual high or low, you may be able to prevent it the next time. Understanding how diabetes works in your child can help to give you the confidence you need to try to solve problems as they arise. It still takes energy and motivation to keep on top of diabetes management, but with education and support, you and your child will learn to live successfully with diabetes.

EXPLAINING DIABETES TO YOUR CHILD

Now that you have a better understanding of highs, lows, targets, goals, and an overview of diabetes, you might be wondering how to explain diabetes to your child. There are excellent resources for children to learn about high and low blood glucose: www.childrenwithdiabetes.com or www.learningdiabetes.com. (See additional resources in resource section, page 201.)

The key to explaining diabetes to your child is to use "teachable" moments. For example, if his blood glucose number is not where you want it to be, discuss with him what the reason might be. Working together with your child is key. Involve him in the conversation and try not to be accusatory or blame your child if a blood glucose is high or low, otherwise he will be on the defensive. You want him to learn from the experience and understand that he will need to take care of himself or else he won't feel well.

TREATING DIABETES TODAY

Diabetes management has come a long way in recent years. From the introduction of blood glucose meters to the development of insulin pumps, pens, and continuous glucose monitoring (discussed in Chapters 3 and 4), taking care of diabetes is easier than ever and will continue to improve the lives of kids with diabetes. Some of the new glucose meters are so easy to use that a young child can learn to do her own tests, although supervision is still essential.

> "A meal plan that's healthy for your child with diabetes is healthy for your whole family. That means everyone can eat the same meals."

Rigid diets are a thing of the past when it comes to managing diabetes. Today, we know that diabetes can be successfully managed with a flexible approach to eating. There are still guidelines and structure to the meal plans, but your child can eat a variety of foods, including some with sugar. Balancing food, insulin, and exercise; testing glucose regularly; and making adjustments when necessary will help your child include special treats in her meal plan.

Science has created new products that make diabetes easier to manage. The development of artificial sweeteners means that children with diabetes can enjoy sweet-tasting foods and drinks without raising blood glucose too high. Insulin has been developed that is much less likely to cause an allergic response than those of the past. Better, more comfortable, shorter and thinner needles, pen devices, and insulin pumps help make giving injections easier.

CHAPTER 2:
Caring For Your Child

Chapter 2:
Caring For Your Child

Having diabetes can affect many aspects of your child's life and your life as a family. Most of the day-to-day care of a child with diabetes is carried out by family members and by the child when he is old enough. In many cases, the burden of care falls on one parent. It is usually best in the beginning to decide as a family how to share responsibilities between family members so that no one person is overloaded. If you are a single parent, you may want to try to enlist help from friends, neighbors, other family members, or churches. Help is essential and you might need to spend some time finding assistance (learn to ask) so that you do not burn out.

PLANNING YOUR CHILD'S CARE

Childcare traditionally tends to fall to mothers. Even in a two-parent family, most of the responsibility will often become hers. It is important for both parents to share responsibilities so that both are knowledgeable about diabetes and involved in your child's care. Work out a system of sharing blood glucose monitoring at night, record keeping, making insulin adjustments, maintaining supplies, and cooking. Siblings are often eager to be involved and can be extremely helpful. Make it a family affair.

When you are deciding on a plan of care with your health care provider, it is important to take into account your child's personality, likes and dislikes, and habits. No two children with diabetes are alike or should be treated in exactly the same way. Obviously, there are some decisions that must be made for safety issues, because it is of utmost importance that he be safe. Otherwise, you can decide together who needs to know, who does not, and how school and social situations can be discreetly and safely handled!

Although many parents at times feel enslaved to the diabetes schedule, it works best if you can plan to fit diabetes care casually into your daily life. Each child with diabetes will have a treatment plan designed for him and his family's schedule. If you and your family, like many, do not have much structure or schedule, it is going to be important to try to organize so that meals can generally be at certain times, sleep schedule is similar from day to day, and insulin times are regular. If you can keep to within about an hour of a usual schedule, you then have a two hour "window" of flexibility from one day to another that will help to keep blood glucose levels steady and predictable. This is a goal, for most days. When weekends, sports, special events, or schedule disruptions occur, you have a base from which to make changes. It will never work perfectly, so be forgiving when you are off-schedule, and move on.

"No two children with diabetes are alike or should be treated in exactly the same way."

The goal of treatment is to keep your child's blood glucose levels within a target range by keeping a three-way balance among insulin, food, and exercise. A treatment plan should include:

- ♦ insulin delivery (injection or pump)
- ♦ blood glucose testing
- ♦ meal planning/food plan

In this triangle of balance one or two sides of the triangle must work to balance a change in the third side.

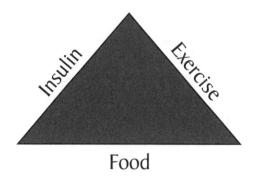

Understanding Your Target Range

You and your health care providers will work together to help you and your child:

♦ Have the best possible control of blood glucoses
♦ Adopt a healthy attitude about living with diabetes at school, at sports, and socially
♦ Deal positively with diabetes within your family.

In 1993, an enormous nine-year study, the Diabetes Control and Complications Trial (DCCT), ended and changed the direction of diabetes care. This very important study clearly showed that keeping blood glucose levels normal or as close to normal as possible can postpone or prevent complications that are caused by diabetes. However, the study had been done with older teens and adults, and we did not know whether we could apply what was learned to children. Many physicians thought that it was better to keep blood glucose levels high in order to avoid the risks of hypoglycemia, and thus there was disagreement among professionals about the goals of treating children with diabetes.

Continuing research shows that keeping blood glucose levels in your child's target range might make a difference in preventing the long-term complications of diabetes. Although low blood glucose levels should be avoided, there seems to be a few long-term effects from having occasional, mild, easily treated hypoglycemia. It is generally agreed that a child's target blood glucose should be as close to normal as possible without risking frequent or severe hypoglycemia. How that happens is widely different from one child to another, and even one physician to another in the same setting. It will depend on how easily blood glucose levels are controlled, the frequency and severity of previous episodes of low blood glucose levels, the type of insulin regimen used, and the stability of the home/school situation.

Tight glucose control—trying to keep glucose levels as close to normal as possible at all times—is not usually recommended for very young children because they are unable to tell someone when they feel symptoms of hypoglycemia. A 2-year-old may not be able to tell you when he feels low; therefore, trying to keep his glucose level in the normal range may cause frequent or severe episodes of hypoglycemia.

A blood glucose goal for a child under 6 years old is generally higher than for older children if the child doesn't report their low blood glucose symptoms. Care must be individualized.

Diabetes health care providers agree that improving blood glucose control is good for everyone with diabetes, including children. The long-term problems that come with high blood glucose levels occur rarely in children, but damage can occur that shows up later in life from behind-the scenes damage to organs and blood vessels. The DCCT study showed that normal blood glucose levels could be achieved through close supervision by a medical team, multiple daily injections or an insulin pump, careful meal planning, meticulous attention to monitoring, and frequent adjustments. It is very important to keep working to get control as good as it can be. You will not be perfect at it, but try not to give up! It's important to try to keep your child's blood glucose within a target range, and to set realistic blood glucose goals for your child.

Develop a Treatment Plan

Developing a treatment plan that meets your child's individual needs, including his eating habits, activity level, and schedule, can help to keep blood glucose levels within the target range. Children and teenagers who do well with their diabetes management seem to follow these practices:

♦ they eat reasonably, consistently, and regularly

♦ they (or their parents) make insulin adjustments and accommodations readily based on their blood glucose levels, schedule, and activities

♦ they test blood glucose levels frequently.

If your child is doing well on his current treatment plan, there may be no need to change anything. But if you and your child are struggling with control issues, you may want to talk with your diabetes health care provider about making changes in the management plan.

WORKING WITH YOUR HEALTH CARE TEAM

One of the lessons of previous research is that people who work closely with a group of health care providers were more successful at managing their diabetes than people who did not. The advantage of working with a health care team is that you have easy access to several different kinds of help. Health care teams usually work in big hospitals or diabetes centers.

Doctors, nurse practitioners, and physician assistants who specialize in diabetes work with you to determine the kind of insulin(s) that will work best for your child, considering her age and your lifestyle. They also determine the dose and regimen that works best for your child, and evaluate your child with a physical exam. A physician specialist in diabetes is called a diabetologist or endocrinologist.

Diabetes educators, who are nurses, dietitians, pharmacists, or other health care professionals, can teach you most of the skills you will need to control your child's diabetes and help you learn how to balance food, exercise, and insulin. In some settings, diabetes nurse educators will provide guidance when you need to adjust insulin doses.

Certified Diabetes Educators (CDE) are licensed health care professionals, such as nurses, dietitians, pharmacists, or exercise physiologists who have taken an exam that verifies that they have met a standard of knowledge about diabetes care and education.

A dietitian will teach you about meal planning and nutrition, help you develop a meal plan based on the food preferences of your child, teach you how to handle holidays and parties, and advise you about the special food needs that children with diabetes have. The dietitian will also suggest ways to increase or decrease calories in a healthy way, based on your child's needs. Dietitians are also often a part of the Certified Diabetes Educator group.

A social worker may help you, your child, and your family deal with concerns about living with diabetes and family issues. Social services can help provide resources for family therapy, finances, parenting skills, and school concerns.

A psychologist or psychiatrist might be part of your team to help you and your child cope with rough times.

There are many issues to deal with in the care of children with diabetes. It is difficult for most primary care providers to keep up on new treatment strategies and new technologies. Therefore, if it is possible for you to go to a center that focuses on pediatric diabetes, it is usually the best way to keep your child in the best blood glucose control possible, and receive the support you need.

If you live a long way from a health care team, you may need to go to your local family doctor or pediatrician for your child's diabetes care. Sometimes, this doctor might suggest that you go to a diabetes center for a diabetes check-up once or twice a year. Your doctor may refer you to other health care providers in your community who can advise you about meal planning, school schedules, insulin adjustments, and coping with stress. It is important that someone experienced and knowledgeable about the treatment of childhood diabetes follows your child's health and that she be seen every three months.

KEEP YOUR CHILD'S BEST INTERESTS AT HEART

The number one player on the health care team is, of course, your child. Your child's physical, mental, and emotional needs are the primary concern of the team. When working with your health care providers (or with other adults in positions of authority, such as teachers at your child's school), you are your child's advocate. You know your child better than anyone. No one else understands his lifestyle, personality, likes, and dislikes as well as you do.

Share what you know about your child openly and honestly with your health care providers, caregivers, and your child's teachers. Your child will benefit from your active participation in decisions about his daily care. If your child is able to assist in the decision-making process, that is even better. Giving him choices will help him feel in control and he might be less likely to argue with your decisions. Sometimes your child will have a creative solution to solve a problem that you might not have even thought of!

The dietitian included fat-free (skim) milk in 4-year-old Andy's meal plan, but Andy doesn't like milk. Andy's mother knew he would never drink the milk and that it would be a battle for everyone if he had to drink it. She explained the problem honestly to the dietitian. Having this information enabled the dietitian to change Andy's meal plan, replacing the milk with liquids that Andy liked and including yogurt for his afternoon snack, which replaced the milk and calcium in his diet. This made it easier for both Andy and his mom to follow the meal plan.

Your child depends on you to support him and to speak on his behalf. Very young children often cannot communicate their needs to adults. Older children may have difficulty expressing their real feelings to adults whom they do not want to disappoint.

Twelve-year-old Missy knew how to give her own insulin injections, but on school mornings when she was in a hurry, she relied on her parents to give her insulin. Missy dreaded going for her diabetes checkups because the doctor always encouraged her to give all her own injections. Missy felt like the doctor didn't understand, but she didn't express her feelings to anyone. Finally, when she told her dad what was bothering her, her dad agreed to talk to the doctor. Together, Missy, her dad, and the doctor agreed on a plan. On school mornings, Missy's mom and dad would alternate giving her insulin injections. In the evenings and on weekends, Missy would do all of her own injections. She learned that honest communication works best, that her dad would be her advocate, and that the doctor would negotiate if he understood the problem.

Make sure that the goals set for your child's diabetes care are realistic, both for him and for you. Goals should be agreed on by everyone. If you or your child cannot meet an expectation or guideline, it is best to tell your diabetes team upfront and honestly. Often, there is another strategy that can be found that addresses the issue.

Fifteen-year-old Joel, who had diabetes since he was 8, knew he should test his blood glucose four times a day, but he disliked the finger sticks. On a good day, he did two blood tests. When Joel wanted to apply for his driver's license, his doctor said that she needed to assess Joel's diabetes control and know that he was taking responsibility for his diabetes before signing the application. To make the assessment, the doctor needed more blood tests from Joel. Together, Joel, his mother, and the doctor set a goal. Joel would test his blood glucose four or more times a day for one month and record the results. At the end of the month, the three of them would look at the test results to assess Joel's diabetes control. Joel was willing to do this because it took him a step closer to getting something he really wanted—his driver's license. (See additional information on driving with diabetes on page 158.)

As a parent, you may need to educate others involved in your child's life. Often those unfamiliar with type 1 diabetes have many misconceptions and misunderstandings about it.

Eight-year-old Amanda loved to go to school and be with her friends. Soon after Amanda was diagnosed with diabetes, her mom noticed she was coming home from school quiet and withdrawn. On her volunteer day at the school, Amanda's mom discovered why: Amanda's classmates seemed to be avoiding her. Amanda's mom asked to speak with the class the next day and brought in a teddy bear, a juice box, and a bottle of insulin. She explained diabetes to the children, showed them the teddy bear needed juice or insulin to feel better, and stressed that no one could catch diabetes from Amanda. Then Amanda showed them how she tested her blood glucose and the kids all asked if they could try it. (The answer was "no"—not without parental permission.) Afterward, the situation smoothed out considerably and Amanda began to play with her friends again.

CHAPTER 3:
Nitty-Gritty I—Insulin

Chapter 3:
Nitty-Gritty I—Insulin

Everyone who has type 1 diabetes needs insulin because there is not enough being made by the pancreas. Insulin must be taken by injection or pump so that it is delivered into the tissue and absorbed into the bloodstream, where it travels to all parts of the body. If insulin would be taken by mouth, it would be digested like protein and wouldn't have any effect on blood glucose levels. Insulin is normally injected into the fatty tissue under the skin.

TYPES OF INSULIN

The first insulins developed came mostly from cows and pigs. These days, the process used to create insulin is "recombinant DNA," which means that insulin is engineered to be exactly like human insulin, yet it is made in a laboratory. It is widely available, can be made in large quantities, and causes fewer allergic reactions than animal insulin. Different kinds of insulin work differently in terms of length of action and peak times (see page 28). The onset is when the insulin starts working, peak time is the period of time when it's working hardest, and duration is how long the insulin lasts.

If your child is doing well on her current insulin, there may be no need to change the type of insulin she uses. If not, you may want to talk to your doctor about different combinations of insulin doses or how she takes her insulin. Insulin can be delivered to the body in many different ways but the usual ways for children are syringes, pens, and pumps. Many diabetes health professionals do not recommend insulin pumps immediately at diagnosis unless the child is a baby or toddler (see page 50). As you go, you can expect that the way your child takes insulin will change based on her age and need for ease of use. Insurance companies

Types of Insulin

There are four types of insulin that work for different lengths of time: rapid-acting, short-acting, intermediate-acting, and long-acting insulins. (For brand names, see the chart on page 30.) You and your health care team will work together to figure out which combination of insulins work best for you.

♦ Rapid-acting (lispro, aspart, glulisine) insulin begins to work almost immediately after being injected. It starts to work in about 5 minutes (onset). It works hardest for an hour or two after injection (this is called the peak). It may last up to about 4–5 hours after injection It is taken right before meals. This insulin works best to handle high blood glucose after eating.

♦ Short-acting (regular) insulin starts to work within half an hour after the injection is given. Regular insulin is usually given 30–45 minutes before a meal and it peaks about 3–4 hours after injection. It can keep working for as long as 6 hours after injection. It is used infrequently but is still valuable in special circumstances.

♦ Intermediate-acting (NPH) insulin works more slowly and usually lasts for 10–16 hours. It may take 30 minutes to 1 hour to begin working and will peak in 4–10 hours after injection. Intermediate-acting insulin is cloudy in the bottle. This type of insulin is often given in the morning and evening but its use is declining in favor of newer products.

♦ Long-acting (glargine or detemir) insulin works for 24 hours after injected, and does not peak (think of it like a marathon runner). These insulins start working in 2–4 hours and can stay in the body for 24 hours with little or no peak. It is injected once or twice a day. This insulin is often called "basal" insulin because it is replacing what the body needs between meals and through the night.

often dictate the brands of products and types of devices that can be used in your plan. It isn't a good idea to switch insulin types, brands, or delivery systems without talking to your doctor or diabetes educator about it first. Review your child's delivery system with your diabetes care provider about every year or so as your child's needs change as he gets older and more capable.

Insulin allergy is very rare; however, if your child has redness or itching at the needle site, you may need to change the insulin type, or the delivery system used. Some parents have reported allergies to the material that helps the syringe to be injected comfortably.

HANDLING INSULIN SAFELY

It's a good idea to keep bottles of insulin in the refrigerator (in the butter keeper or somewhere else where it will not freeze). Insulin can break down and not work if it gets too cold (below 36°F) or too warm (over 86°F). Never store insulin near extreme heat or extreme cold.

You can also store insulin at room temperature or carry it with you in a purse, pocket, or backpack. Airport x-ray machines do not hurt insulin when you are traveling. An opened bottle of insulin is stable at room temperature for up to 28 days, as long as it is stored away from heat and light. If your child uses up a bottle of insulin in less than a month, it's okay to keep it at room temperature. If she uses small amounts of insulin, it is generally recommended that you discard the unused portion 28 days after being opened. Mark the date on the bottle when you open it so that you can track it. It's a good idea to keep the bottle in the carton to protect it from light and keep it clean.

Some people prefer to keep insulin in the refrigerator and take it out for a few minutes to warm up before giving the injection. Others don't seem to notice if the insulin is cool when injected.

How to Dispose of Needles

It's important to handle and dispose of used needles and lancets safely. It's safest not to recap needles or lancets. This helps you avoid being accidentally stuck. Your diabetes educator may be able to either provide

Insulins Used in the U.S.

Generic	Brand Name	Form	Manufacturer
Rapid-acting			
insulin glulisine	Apidra	analog	Sanofi-Aventis
insulin lispro	Humalog	analog	Eli Lilly
insulin aspart	NovoLog	analog	Novo Nordisk
Regular			
regular	Humulin R	human	Eli Lilly
regular	Novolin R	human	Novo Nordisk
Intermediate-acting			
NPH	Humulin N	human	Eli Lilly
NPH	Novolin N ReliOn (Walmart)	human	Novo Nordisk
Long-acting			
insulin detemir	Levemir	analog	Novo Nordisk
insulin glargine	Lantus	analog	Sanofi-Aventis
Mixtures			
70% NPH/30% regular	Humulin 70/30	human	Eli Lilly
70% NPH/30% regular	Novolin 70/30	human	NovoNordisk
50% lispro protamine/ 50% insulin lispro	Humalog mix 50/50	analog	Eli Lilly
75% lispro protamine (NPL)/25% lispro	Humalog mix 75/50	analog	Eli Lilly
70% aspart protamine/ 30% aspart	Humalog mix 70/30	analog	Novo Nordisk

you with or suggest where you can find a special box to use for disposing of needles and lancets (called a "Sharps box"). Some pharmacies carry them. Otherwise, use a plastic milk carton or a soda or detergent bottle. Check with your local trash disposal company township or borough to find out how to label and dispose of the used needle container in your community.

HOW MUCH INSULIN DOES MY CHILD NEED?

Insulin dosages are based on your child's height, weight, metabolism, physical maturity, activity level, and meal plan. A heavier or taller child usually needs more insulin than a smaller child, and a child who isn't active may need more insulin than one who is. A teen going through puberty might need significantly more insulin than a school-age child. A newly diagnosed child might need very small amounts.

For a few months after a child is diagnosed with diabetes, she may need only a very low dose of insulin. During this period, which is sometimes called the "honeymoon period," the child's pancreas still produces some insulin. As time goes by, the insulin-producing beta cells are destroyed. As these cells produce less and less insulin, your child will need more insulin.

One 12-year-old child may take a daily dose of 60 units while another takes 45 and another takes only 20 units. Taking a larger dose of insulin doesn't mean the child's diabetes is more severe.

> "Needing to increase the insulin dose does not mean your child's diabetes is getting worse."

Needing to increase the dose does not mean your child's diabetes is getting worse. Different dosages simply mean that children are different, and their bodies have different requirements.

Your child's need for insulin may change from one year to the next, one season to the next, and sometimes one day to the next. This is why it is important to monitor her glucose level frequently so that you can determine your child's insulin needs. Reviewing patterns of blood glucose (either on paper, a meter, or continuous glucose monitor) is essential to help determine when changes need to be made. Generally, as children grow, they need more insulin. Many children need more insulin in winter than in summer because of differences in their activity level. In winter, kids are often less active, are in school, and are indoors more, whereas in the summer they may spend more time playing outside.

Big changes in your child's insulin dosage should only be made after discussion with your doctor or diabetes educator, but fine-tuning your child's dosage from day to day is something you can and should learn to do yourself (see page 43). Most diabetes pediatric teams have a diabetes educator who can help you if you are uncertain about what to change, or if the changes you have made are not working.

HOW OFTEN DOES MY CHILD NEED INJECTIONS?

We know from research that the best way of managing diabetes is to precisely match insulin to food and exercise. The best way to do this is to match your child's insulin to how he eats. A long-acting basal (or "background") insulin dose works slowly and gives the body a steady, low level of insulin to manage blood glucose levels between meals. Basal insulin mimics the body's natural low-level steady background release of insulin. Use basal insulin along with rapid-acting (bolus) insulin that covers meals and covers high blood glucose levels. Bolus insulin is an extra amount of insulin taken to cover an expected rise in blood glucose. This regimen is called "basal/bolus" or multiple daily injections (MDI) and can be done with syringes, pens, or pumps. It works for all ages. It mimics the way a normal pancreas works, releasing bursts of insulin after each meal and maintaining a 24-hour long-acting insulin level to keep the blood glucose stable between meals and through the night.

Today's comfortable needles for rapid-acting insulin make an MDI plan quite safe and feasible for children. Basal-bolus regimens through MDI or pumps provide a bit more flexibility: the insulin dosage can be adjusted frequently during the day according to food intake and activity level. (For more about pump therapy, see page 46.)

Children and teens are encouraged to use basal/bolus insulin regimens because that is the best way to match insulin, food, and

Daily Injections

Children and teens control diabetes with a minimum of three injections a day. The number of daily injections your child needs is based on:

♦ the type of insulin your child takes

♦ how motivated your child is to care for her diabetes herself

♦ the quality of family and other support available

♦ your child's level of blood glucose control

♦ your child's schedule, exercise level, and meal plan

♦ patterns of blood glucose that emerge with frequent monitoring

♦ the types of insulin used

exercise. A basal/bolus approach also helps to address a need for flexibility in schedules and variable appetites. You have more flexibility in your meal times, can eat different portions of food, and will learn to adjust insulin accordingly. However, if the teen skips many of the injections, he may need to step back to a less intensive but easier regimen to ensure that he gets all the insulin he needs.

To avoid gaps or overlaps between doses, a good rule of thumb is to give the injections at regular times, within about an hour of the target time. Basal/bolus insulin works best when life gets off-schedule because the basal insulin works for 24 hours, and you can take your rapid-acting insulin when you eat. During summer vacation, holidays, or any other time when your child's schedule changes, it's okay to gradually alter the times of meals, snacks, and insulin injections. For example, if your child wants to get up and eat breakfast later during the summer months, the whole schedule can be pushed back. Your doctor or diabetes educator can help you and your child decide how to handle these kinds of schedule changes.

Scheduling Meals and Insulin Injections

A helpful rule of thumb is to give injections and have meals about the same time (give or take an hour). Although basal/bolus insulin plans are intended to provide flexibility, these plans work better when you at least try to follow a general schedule. If your child takes an insulin such as NPH—which has a peak action time, it is even more important to eat on time. Here's how this might work.

♦ Usual wake up time: 7 a.m.

   Give the injection of breakfast insulin before breakfast (between 6 and 8 a.m.).

♦ Usual lunch time: noon

   Eat lunch no earlier than 11 a.m. and no later than 1 p.m. If your child takes rapid-acting insulin, try to give the injection immediately before lunch, unless your child's blood glucose is <80 mg/dl and she has to stand in a cafeteria line and lunch could be delayed. In such a case, she could take her insulin pen to the cafeteria, if the school district allows it, to take the injection with her food. A less than ideal alternative would be to take the insulin after she eats.

♦ Usual dinner time: 5 p.m.

   Eat dinner no earlier than 4 p.m. and no later than 6 p.m. Give the injection of rapid-acting insulin immediately before eating, or immediately afterward in a young child with a variable appetite.

♦ Usual bed time: 9:30 p.m.

   Give long-acting insulin before bedtime snack (if your child eats a bedtime snack). If not, you may need rapid-acting insulin to correct for a high blood glucose level.

GIVING THE INJECTIONS

Giving your child an insulin injection can be hard, both emotionally and physically, especially if your child is young and squirms a lot. It is always a good idea to prepare the syringes first before calling your young child, especially if he is a squirmer. This way, he won't have to wait so long and may be less anxious. The material presented here may give you some guidance.

- Hold the syringe like a pencil and insert the needle gently at a 90° angle to the skin (straight up and down).
- Push gently but steadily on the plunger.
- Give the injection quickly or slowly, depending on your child's preference.
- Pull the needle out and throw it immediately (uncapped) into a proper disposal container (a "sharps box").
- After the injection, praise your child for doing a good job and give her a big hug.

Insulin syringes are now shorter and finer than ever, and in most cases, it is not necessary to pinch up the skin. The only time pinching is suggested is in a very lean, muscular child or a baby. Ask your diabetes educator if you should pinch up the skin or not, if you are uncertain. Injecting the insulin into a muscle can be painful and can also alter the way insulin is absorbed. Some children report that the short syringes hurt more, possibly because the depth of penetration is closer to nerves on the surface. (The proper method for drawing up insulin is found in the Appendix in the back, page 189.)

WHAT IS SITE ROTATION?

It is important to give your child's insulin injections in different places. Rotating insulin injection sites and insulin pump sites is important so that puffy, lumpy spots do not develop and hinder the absorption of insulin. When insulin is injected in the same site over time, it might attract fat into the injection area, leading to the formation of lumps made of fat and scar tissue. Absorption of insulin from these areas is poor. Injecting into these lumps will delay the absorption of insulin and blood glucose levels will be difficult to manage.

Making a plan for rotating injections is beneficial because it can help you and your child remember which site to use for a specific insulin injection. For example, if your child gets multiple injections a day, you could give the morning injection in the abdomen, lunch injection in the arm, dinner injection in the leg, and the evening long-acting injection in the hip. Using a rotation schedule such as this will help you remember which site you should be using for a specific time of day.

You may also want to rotate within one area—like the fleshy part of the upper arm—by dividing it with imaginary lines (see Appendix on page 192). Different spots of the body have different rates of absorption. Generally speaking, a very muscular area will have more rapid absorption than a fatty area. A limb such as an arm or leg that is moving or exercising can have increased absorption because of the increased blood flow to the limb. Insulin is absorbed most quickly when the injection is given in the abdomen. It is absorbed a bit more slowly when the injection is given in the arms, more slowly in the legs, and slowest of all when the injection is given in the hip. Larger amounts of insulin are usually most comfortable when given in the hip or abdomen.

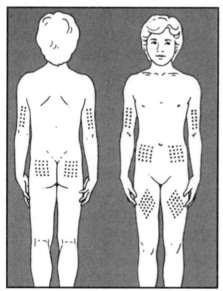

Injection sites for children

If your child is having wide swings in blood glucose levels, keep track of the injection sites you are using. This can help you see if the swings have a pattern that is related to the injection site. (For example, do your child's blood glucose levels swing more when the injections are given in the hip than when they are given in the arms?) Your diabetes educator can help you and your child decide on the best way to do site rotation.

HELPING YOUR CHILD ACCEPT INJECTIONS

Every child responds differently to the intrusion of injections. Some children adjust well to insulin injections, while others find them very hard to accept. There are several reasons why a child may fight injections.

- ◆ The injection may be painful or there may be past associations of pain with injections.
- ◆ The child may be expressing anger about having diabetes.
- ◆ Your child might actually think the pricks are a form of punishment for being "bad."
- ◆ The child may be afraid of needles.
- ◆ It may be an age-related problem. (Preschool children generally do not do well with any kind of intrusive procedure.)

Very young children may fuss during injections. It may help to tell your child that the injection keeps her healthy and to give her a big hug when it's over. The fuss usually subsides over time as your child becomes used to getting injections regularly.

To get your child used to the idea of getting insulin injections, it may help in the beginning to associate the injection with something the child enjoys, like watching a favorite show on television. Say, "Every day, just before you watch XYZ show, mom (or dad) will give you your insulin to keep you well." It is generally not suggested that you give an injection to your child when he is sleeping. The bed should be a "safe" place. If you need to inject your sleeping child, it is best to arouse him enough to announce what you are going to do. Most of the time your child won't fully awaken, and probably will not remember it in the morning.

In families where both parents are available, it's a good idea for both to be involved in giving the child's insulin injections. That way, both parents share the responsibility and one parent does not always feel like the bad guy. Also, try to avoid the word "shot." Although commonly used, this word can mean shot with a gun or arrow to children.

If your child is having a hard time with the injections, you might also try putting ice on the skin prior to the injection, or a topical anesthetic such as Bactine or Solarcaine. There is also a topical anesthetic called

Emla cream, which is a prescription that some physicians will prescribe before blood work. If your child has a hard time with changing pump sites, it can be applied to the skin at the new infusion site about two hours before the site is changed for maximum effectiveness.

If the child is complaining about the pain from an injection, there is usually a reason. An injection may be more painful than usual if: it is given in dense muscle tissue, it caused a bruise, the injection was given close to a nerve ending, or the needle is slightly bent or blunted when the insulin is withdrawn from the bottle. Consult your doctor or diabetes educator if your child frequently complains of pain during injections. However, many children complain more at the idea of having the injection than because the injection itself is actually painful.

It's normal for children to protest about injections at times, especially when they are tired, stressed, or unhappy. However, if your family's life is consistently disrupted by your child's resistance to injections, a social worker or psychologist may be able to help with the transition. Often, the child just wants to be heard! In other words, she is protesting that she has diabetes, doesn't want to have to do this, and wants you to be considerate of that fact.

GIVING THEIR OWN INJECTIONS

Learning to give their own injections is an important step for children with diabetes because it helps them be more independent. They can go to visit relatives or on sleepovers with friends. Most important, they can feel in charge of their diabetes.

There is no strict age when children are ready to start giving their own injections. One child may be ready to do it (with a parent watching) at age 7, while another child may not be ready until age 11. The right age for your child is whenever she is capable of doing it and when both you and the child feel comfortable about her doing it.

Try to be patient and let your child do the injections when she feels ready, but remind her that you are always there to help. She may quickly get the hang of giving her own injections and may do it without your help for a while. Then, for some reason, she may again want you to help

Tips for Easier Insulin Injections

If you are worried that the injection hurts your child:

♦ Try an injection on yourself! Inject yourself in the arm or abdomen with a syringe to see what the needle feels like. (Do not inject anything into the skin.) You may be relieved to find that it hardly hurts because the needle is so fine.

If your child wants to give her own injection in the arm:

♦ Have her press her arm against a chair or a wall or over a bent knee to help to make the fleshy part of the arm stand out.

If insulin frequently leaks out after you give the injection:

♦ This happens most often to a lean or muscular person. Try pulling the skin to one side when pinching it up.

♦ After pushing in the plunger, count slowly to 10 before removing the needle.

If the plunger won't push in easily:

♦ Pull back slightly on the needle. If the plunger still won't move easily, take the needle out and try giving the injection at another spot. If the plunger still won't move, fill a new syringe and start over. The insulin may be jamming the needle.

If your child gets bruising around the area of the injection:

♦ Bruising is usually caused by a small broken blood vessel. It's hard to avoid bruising once in a while. Unless it happens a lot, it isn't something to worry about. If it does happen a lot, ask your diabetes educator for help with your injection technique.

If the area of the injection turns red:

♦ Redness may be caused by alcohol that is used to clean the skin or sometimes the silicone or other substance used on the syringe needle to make it insert smoothly. If alcohol irritates your child's skin, use soap and water instead. Rarely, redness may be caused by an allergic reaction to insulin.

or to give the injection. It is common for children to move forward and then step back. You may wonder why you need to do it for her since she can do it herself, but kids may need your help for a while. Sometimes they need reassurance that they can still rely on their parents' support.

Your child may feel okay about giving injections in the legs but not in the arms or abdomen. You may need to keep doing those injections for a while. You may want to suggest that you give the injections on odd-numbered days and that your child gives them on even-numbered days.

"Try to be patient and let your child do the injections when she feels ready, but remind her that you are there to help."

Wanting to go on a camping trip or sleepover at a friend's house may give your child an incentive to learn to do her own injections. Getting to know other children who can give their own injections may also help. Encourage your child to attend a youth group or a camp for children with diabetes. Don't be surprised if a letter home from camp announces with pride, "I gave my own injection today!"

Even when you feel comfortable about your child giving her own injections, supervision is always recommended. A responsible adult should check to make sure the dose is correct and that all the insulin is injected. Children (even teenagers) always feel more secure when their parents are involved in their diabetes care (although teens might not act that way). Kids also wax and wane on what they do, and although they are often physically able to give their own injections, and may have even been independent doing it for a while, they often will quit unless you are monitoring and supervising them.

ADJUSTING INSULIN AT HOME

Your child's insulin requirement and doses will vary from day to day. With help from your health care provider, you will learn how to make small adjustments in your child's daily insulin dosage depending on what she has to eat and how active she is. Major changes in your child's insulin

Encourage Your Child To Give Injections

Encourage your child one step at a time.

1. Start by asking your child to choose the injection site, and wipe it off with soap and water, or alcohol.

2. Have her just lay her hand over yours when you give it, so she can feel the movement.

3. Have her hold the syringe, with your hand on top of hers while you give the injection.

4. With your hand still on top, have her give the injection.

5. Let her try putting the needle in on her own.

6. She should work at putting the needle in and pushing down on the plunger.

Give your child lots of praise as she takes on greater responsibility for injections. Eventually, your child will be able to do the whole procedure herself!

dose should only be made with the guidance of your doctor or diabetes educator; however, you can make small changes (within 10% of the usual dose) yourself when you are comfortable doing so.

Fine-tuning your child's dosage helps to keep her blood glucose levels in the target range. Looking for patterns in glucose levels will help you adjust the insulin dose. Record keeping is very important. Without good documentation of what is going on, it is almost impossible to figure out what changes need to be made. Most of today's blood glucose meters have an internal memory along with the ability to upload data into a computer; however, keeping daily logs is still one of the most important tasks in managing diabetes.

Remember that neither the amount of insulin nor the number of injections your child needs is a measure of the severity of her diabetes. As your child grows, she will need more insulin. Growth hormones— epinephrine, cortisol, glucagon, and all of the hormones of puberty— cause insulin needs to increase. If there is not enough insulin present during times of growth, she may not grow well. As your child grows and needs more insulin, it doesn't mean his diabetes has gotten worse—he's just gotten bigger!

How Food and Exercise Affect Insulin Needs

The amount of insulin your child needs from day to day is based upon how much and what type of food she eats and how active she is. Your diabetes educator can help you learn how to make daily adjustments to your child's insulin dosage depending on the food and activities planned for that day.

Food raises blood glucose while exercise usually lowers it. Eating more than usual or eating a sugar-rich food like birthday cake can make your child's blood glucose rise. Taking part in a strenuous game can make it drop.

James, who is 8 years old, is going on an overnight scout camping trip. When James is camping, his glucose level is usually in his target range because of all the games and activities. But the troop plans to roast marshmallows and make popcorn at the campfire. James doesn't really understand counting carbohydrates, so he doesn't know how much he can eat.

James wants to eat the marshmallows with his friends, but they will probably raise his blood glucose. His mom suggests that he test his blood glucose before the campfire. She tells him that his blood sugar will probably be okay from all of the games played that evening. She consults with a dietitian about carbohydrates, and they come up with a plan. She writes the following note for James:

Dear James,
Enjoy 4 to 6 cups of popcorn! And . . . .
Eat 6 marshmallows if your blood test is less than 80.
Eat 4 marshmallows if your blood test is 80 to 180.
Eat 2 marshmallows if your blood test is over 180.
Love, Mom

Extra food helps to balance exercise. When your child plans to exercise, you can decrease insulin, give her more food to eat, or both. When blood glucose runs high, you can give more insulin or adjust the child's meal plan so she eats less. If your child is going through a phase when she eats less than usual, she will need less insulin. Your doctor or diabetes educator can help you to understand how to balance food, activity, and insulin to keep your child's blood glucose level in her target range. (See Playing Games and Sports, page 97, and The Nitty-Gritty 3—Meal Plans, page 71, for more on how food and exercise affect your child's need for insulin.)

How Do I Fine-Tune My Child's Dosage?

Fine-tuning your child's insulin dosage means:

♦ learning to look for patterns of high or low blood glucose
♦ trying to figure out why high or low blood glucose levels occur
♦ adjusting your child's insulin dose, food, or timing of meals to fix the problem.

If your child's blood glucose level is a bit too high, you can increase the insulin dose or reduce food. If your child's blood glucose level is a bit too low, you can decrease the dose or add food. When glucose is:

High   ↑   Increase insulin

Low   ↓   Decrease insulin

However, there are some exceptions to this rule (see rebound effect, page 117).

There are various ways to manage diabetes and adjust insulin. One of the more traditional ways is to use a "sliding scale." A sliding scale gives you a fixed dose of insulin based on blood glucose levels. The only way a sliding scale can work well, however, is if the child or teen eats a consistent amount of carbs, fat, and protein at the meal when he gets the insulin. Many kids are very consistent about their meals and will follow a meal plan comprised of healthy food groups. If that is the case for your child, the sliding scale should work.

A Sliding Scale for Rapid-Acting Insulin

Find the blood glucose range in the column on the left. Then look at the column on the right to find the corresponding insulin dose. For example, if Jimmy's blood glucose reading is 142 mg/dl, he should take 5 units of insulin.

Subtract 2 units if your child will be exercising strenuously. For example, if Jimmy's blood glucose reading is 135 mg/dl but he will be playing soccer after breakfast, he should take 3 units of insulin.

Blood glucose reading(mg/dl) (before breakfast)	Insulin dose
<70	3 units
70–120	4 units
121–180	5 units
181–240	6 units
241–300	7 units
>300	8 units

The box above gives an example of how insulin doses can be adjusted according to a blood glucose level. Your doctor or diabetes educator can prepare a dosage adjustment chart or scale that's right for your child.

Why Are Patterns in Blood Glucose Levels Important?

It may take a few days for a dosage adjustment to make a difference in your child's blood glucose control, so it is important to look for patterns in blood glucose levels over periods of three or four days.

Mike had soccer practice from 7 to 8 p.m. on Mondays, Wednesdays, and Fridays. Halfway through practice he would have symptoms of hypoglycemia. To prevent low blood glucose during soccer practice, Mike reduced his before-dinner dose of aspart (rapid-acting) insulin by 50% on soccer nights.

When blood glucose levels aren't where you want them to be, keep a record of what time of day the problem is occurring, as well as any possible reasons you could think of for the high or low numbers. Keeping track can help you and your health care provider decide how to fine-tune your child's dosage. This is why blood glucose testing throughout the day is important. Not only can you see where the problems arise, you can try to fix them.

INSULIN DELIVERY DEVICES

As technology has progressed and multiple daily injections have become more common, the use of insulin pens and insulin pumps has become more popular.

Insulin Pens

For many years, people with diabetes have been interested in devices that will improve insulin injections. The idea of "getting a shot" has been a scary notion. The insulin pen is one invention that has revolutionized the convenience, appearance, and comfort of insulin injections. The insulin pen looks like a pen that you might write with and keep in your pocket, but it has insulin inside. When you are ready to take an injection, you put on a needle, dial up the correct dose, and inject. It's that simple! Along with their easy use, insulin pens are also convenient because people using them don't have to carry insulin bottles and syringes around with them. You just grab the pen and go.

Insulin pens might help with injections in children and teens who are afraid of syringes. A child might also find it easier to put the needle through the skin or to give injections in hard-to-reach places.

Although there have been several styles of pens developed over the past few years—from completely disposable to a permanent pen with a disposable cartridge—most companies are leaning toward disposable pens. Both types are easy to use and have dials to make insulin dosing a snap. Along with the pen, there are disposable needles, of various lengths, that must be changed with each injection. The pens are available from manufacturers in several different types of insulin.

In children, especially young children, one important consideration regarding the use of a pen is to consider whether or not your child needs ½ unit increments when you are measuring insulin. There are only a few types of pens that can measure in ½ units, so be sure to ask your diabetes educator for recommendations if your child requires it.

"Insulin pens might help with injections in children and teens who are afraid of syringes."

Not every type of insulin is available for insulin pen use. Also, you cannot mix types of insulin together in a special ratio. The pens do come already premixed in standard ratios (70/30 NPH/Regular, for example), but the dose cannot be changed as needed, which most children require. Pens are portable, manageable, and the "dial-a-dose" format is easy for kids to do accurately. With the disposable pens, it is now possible for kids to leave one pen at their friend's house, one in school, one at Grandma's, and carry one for spontaneous use at a restaurant!

Insulin Pumps

Another technological advancement has revolutionized diabetes care in the past few years with the invention of the insulin pump. People with diabetes needed a convenient and precise way of balancing insulin, food, and exercise that both controlled blood glucose and matched their lifestyle. Thus, the insulin pump evolved. An insulin pump is a small battery-run device that continually delivers insulin to the body.

The first pumps were used in the 1970's, but they were large and had few safety features. They have grown increasingly smaller, safer, and easier to use. Today's pumps are small, electronically smart, and have many safety features and alerts to make diabetes management easier than ever. They can very precisely deliver small amounts of insulin—an important feature for young children who need very small doses. All pumps have the ability to know how much insulin to give in response to carbohydrates eaten.

The pump is either connected to a flexible catheter (straw) or directs

Tips for Insulin Pen Use

1. Make sure the pen that you receive can measure ½ unit increments if your child needs them. Some pens only measure 1 unit at a time, which might not work for a small child.
2. Change needle tips with every use.
3. Make sure that you "prime" the needle tip with insulin so that it is ready to deliver when you insert it. (There can be dead space where a tiny amount of air remains in the hub of the new needle.) Push insulin through until you see a drop come out of the tip of the needle. By doing this, you will have removed the air so that you do not decrease the dose of insulin you intend to give.
4. Pens tend to deliver insulin slower than a syringe, so you must leave the needle in longer when injecting. Leave the needle in place for 10 seconds so that insulin is not oozing out of the needle when you pull it out of the skin.

an insulin pod to deliver the insulin. The soft, comfortable catheter is inserted into subcutaneous tissue, usually the abdomen or hip and left in place for 2 days. Insulin flows through the needle from the pump or pod. The device itself is about the size of a small cell phone, and stores a supply of rapid-acting insulin. It is worn all the time, but can be disconnected for bathing, swimming, or contact sports. It should not be disconnected for more than an hour at a time.

Using an insulin pump is a form of intensive diabetes management, where the aim is to keep blood glucose levels in your target range as much as possible. The idea of pump therapy is to provide flexibility so that you can respond to changes in blood glucose levels, exercise, or food eaten. Insulin is delivered continually by preprogrammed amounts that can be temporarily or permanently changed as necessary. This is called the "basal" insulin. When the person eats or drinks carbohydrates, or needs insulin to correct a high blood glucose level, the pump will suggest an amount to take, which can be altered if needed. This is called "bolus" insulin, and is the same concept as balas/bolus with injections (see page 32).

Insulin pumps are quite helpful for managing diabetes for children, teens, and especially infants (due to the pumps' ability to deliver extremely small amounts of insulin precisely).

" Even though using an insulin pump has disadvantages, most pump users agree that the advantages outweigh the disadvantages. "

Current pumps are very smart and take away some of the user-variability and responsibility of having to decide doses. Modern pump technology tracks how much insulin has been delivered, when it was delivered, and how much of it is still working in the body, so there's less chance of taking too much or too little and ending up with low or high blood glucose. A parent can look at the history in a menu to see what doses their child took throughout the day, or how many carbohydrates were eaten. Pumps will provide alerts and alarms when the insulin reservoir is low, the battery is low, or there is no delivery.

Although pump therapy is generally safe, and there are alarms on the pump if anything should go wrong, it is easy to develop hyperglycemia if there is a leak or obstruction in the tubing or catheter. Also, keep in mind that with an insulin pump, you are only using rapid-acting insulin. So if there is a problem such as a kink, leak, obstruction, or bad site, your child has no basal insulin, and he can get very sick from a high blood glucose level very quickly. The pump user must be careful about monitoring blood glucose and be prepared to change the infusion site if unexplained high blood glucose should occur. It is also possible to develop infections at the infusion site, although this is unusual if good hygiene practices are followed.

There are pluses and minuses to using a pump. Even though using an insulin pump has disadvantages, most pump users agree the advantages outweigh the disadvantages. Because today's pumps are not yet automatic, and rely on the user to do her part, common sense says that it

Advantages/Disadvantages of Pump Use

Advantages

- Eliminates daily individual insulin injections
- Delivers insulin more accurately than injections
- Often improves AIC
- Usually results in few large swings in blood glucose levels
- Allows your child to be flexible about when and what you eat
- Can improve your child's quality of life
- Reduces severe low blood glucose episodes
- Allows your child to exercise without having to eat large amounts of carbohydrates

Disadvantages

- Can cause weight gain if your child covers extra food with extra insulin
- Can cause diabetic ketoacidosis (DKA) if the catheter comes out and your child doesn't get insulin for hours
- Can be expensive
- Can be bothersome since you are attached to the pump most of the time

is only a tool and like almost any tool, is only as effective as the person using it. In the hands of a motivated, careful user, a pump can be a very helpful and precise way of managing diabetes. In the hands of a user who expects the pump to do the work for him and who may not want to put effort into doing the work, it may be no better than any other method of insulin delivery. Although pump therapy does promote flexibility and convenience, it still takes time, attention, and energy. Pump users must test their blood glucose at least four times a day and be diligent about problem solving. At least at first, it is essential to work closely with a doctor or diabetes educator to decide on insulin dosages or handle any problems that come up.

Most insulin pump companies have software and devices to upload insulin pumps so that all of the information is graphed. The information obtained helps you and your diabetes professional better understand how your child actually uses his pump and could highlight where problems exist.

Is a pump right for my child?
Insulin pumps are great tools for parents and kids when used properly. The use of insulin pump therapy in children is widely accepted. For very young children, it is the only way of precisely delivering extremely small amounts of insulin; however, some children are not developmentally able to handle the responsibility of a pump, so they will need parental administration, like injections. Most school-age kids and teens find the pump more socially acceptable than taking injections. They also find it useful in responding to changing activity, food, and hormone levels.

Using a pump may be an option for a child or teenager who:

♦ needs a more flexible meal plan or freedom from multiple insulin injections
♦ is mature enough to look after the pump and check her blood glucose levels regularly
♦ has support and supervision at home and at school.

For a teen who is mostly responsible for her own decisions, a pump can work very well, if she is motivated to care for her diabetes. Parents should not assume that their child is doing a good job using his pump, even though he is very capable of doing so. For younger children, the responsibility for diabetes care usually falls on the parent, who must continue to supervise and stay involved on a daily basis. If you and your child are interested in using a pump, you should arrange to see a diabetes educator who has experience working with children who use pumps.

Troubleshooting pump issues

One common problem that can occur with pump therapy is a "bad" infusion site. This refers to the portal where insulin enters the body. A small crimp or bend in the tubing, or the needle tip pressed against a muscle fiber or compressed tubing, can cause insulin not to flow.

When your child is using a pump and her blood sugar is running unexpectedly high, the first thing you should do is give a dose to correct the blood sugar and wait an hour. If in one hour, blood glucose is not coming down, it is usually best to change the site, as a bad site is the most common reason for high blood glucose on pumps. Even a modest compression from a belt or from sitting or lying on the needle could affect the flow of insulin. Most diabetes educators and pump trainers recommend changing the tubing and reservoir (or pod) just in case the insulin delivery problem involved the tubing, reservoir, or connections between the various parts. Be prepared to give an injection of insulin until the problem is solved.

Some helpful hints to avoid pumping problems include:

- If you are considering insulin pump therapy for your child, do some homework before beginning the process. Speak to your health care providers, talk to parents and to kids with pumps about their likes and dislikes, and read about the features of the various pumps on manufacturers' websites.

- Everyone should learn about the pump and how to use it. This includes parents, grandparents, and siblings. Be as prepared as possible for your initial pump training and seek out and attend advanced pump classes. With such an expensive instrument, it makes sense to learn to use it to its full advantage!

- It is best to stay on a schedule and change the site every 2 days. Pick even or odd days and stick to it as much as possible. If you let the site change go longer, often by the third day, you will notice that blood glucose levels are running higher. This might be even more obvious in the summer months because heat can interfere with insulin's effectiveness.

- Don't change the site close to bedtime. If you happen to have a site that is not working at bedtime, your child or teen may awaken with large ketones or vomiting by morning. Give yourself the opportunity to recheck blood glucose before sleep.

- Don't forget to fill the cannula (tiny plastic straw left in place) after changing the reservoir, tubing, or pod. When this step is omitted, it can take a few hours for the pump to fill the empty cannula with insulin, and your child will have no insulin going into his tissues until the cannula fills.

- Secure the infusion set so it doesn't pull out. In a sweaty, busy, or active kid it is common for the infusion set to pull out. There are types of sticky skin prep, such as Skin-Tac, that can help adhesive to stick to skin better. This is available through places that sell pumps and through pharmacies and online resources. There are also creative ways for kids to wear their pumps that are more secure, such as inside pockets, cami's, or T-shirts.

- Work with your child to make sure bolus doses are given, and correct. Kids, like adults, can sometimes forget to take their bolus dose. Sometimes they truly forget, while other times it is either not convenient, they think they'll do it later, or are afraid if they do take it, they will be "low" later.

- Ask your physician for suggestions on how to manage if your child will be disconnected for longer periods of time. If your child is involved in sports where disconnecting is advised, it is usually recommended that the child take about an hour's worth of basal insulin (or less) before disconnecting, and not leave the pump off for more than an hour. Disconnecting for more than an hour can lead to high blood glucose levels later on. Children who must be disconnected for even longer periods of time sometimes use long-acting insulin.

- Most low blood glucose levels can be effectively treated by 12–16 grams of glucose, unless your child is exercising. You may find that 30 grams of carbohydrate are necessary when he is exercising. Treatment is based on experience, so keep a log of what you do so you can see what works and what doesn't.

♦ Stay involved in your child's diabetes management. There is a tendency for parents to be less involved with their child's diabetes management when the child is on a pump. It is important for parents to remember that kids and teens need you to stay closely involved in decision-making so that they can do their best. They may not want you to be involved, but they do "need" you to be involved in their care. Do your best to make it a team effort.

Pumps are integrating with continuous glucose monitoring technology in an effort to better maintain normal blood glucose levels. The long-term goal is to develop a mechanical device that can respond to blood glucose levels appropriately and automatically keep them within normal limits as much as possible. This is called a "closed loop" system. Manufacturers and researchers are approaching this goal one step at a time.

CHAPTER 4:
Nitty-Gritty 2—Glucose

Chapter 4:
Nitty-Gritty 2—Glucose

Routine monitoring (testing of blood glucose levels) is a very important part of your child's diabetes care. Glucose readings are done using a meter that measures the amount of glucose in a drop of capillary blood, usually from the finger. Glucose meters are so easy to use that most children can quickly learn how to do their own glucose tests. Continuous glucose monitoring, a technology that also measures blood glucose can also provide glucose information (see page 61). These readings, plus a laboratory test called A1C, are your tools for keeping blood glucose levels in the target range.

WHAT IS AN AIC TEST?

The A1C is a useful blood test that your doctor should do to measure your child's average blood glucose control over a period of 2–3 months. The A1C measures the amount of glycosylated hemoglobin (a form of hemoglobin to which glucose has joined) in your blood. The American Diabetes Association recommends an A1C less than 7% in adults. (See page 12 for goals for children and teens.) Research has shown that keeping your child's A1C within her target range will delay or prevent complications later in life. (See Complications of Diabetes, page 124.)

The A1C is usually taken from blood drawn and read in the lab. Some health care offices and clinics have the machine that can read it from a blood sample taken from your finger. There are also kits to do this that you can buy.

It is important to keep in mind that anything that causes a high blood glucose level, such as an illness or stress, can affect the A1C value. For example, strep throat caused your child's blood glucose levels to be high for a week, so his A1C result is affected. Sometimes life gets in the way of good control, so if your child's test results are higher than you

Calculating Your eAG

If your A1C is (%)	Your eAG is (mg/dl)
5	97
5.5	111
6	126
6.5	140
7	154
7.5	169
8	183
8.5	197
9	212
9.5	226
10	240
10.5	255
11	269
11.5	283
12	298

would like, use this number as a new starting point and work toward an improvement on the next test.

To make the comparison of your blood glucose levels and your A1C easier, your health care providers will probably give you another number with your A1C. This number is called the estimated average glucose (eAG), and is often considered more meaningful because it relates your blood glucose to an average blood glucose number. Instead of getting 7%, it would report as 154 mg/dl, which is easier to translate for people who are used to getting similar numbers on their glucose meter (see Calculating Your eAG, left). The A1C test is a very important part of diabetes care. Make sure that your child is having this test done every three months and that the results are given to you. There are now home A1C tests available. Use these results to guide your adjustments and diabetes management.

DAILY MONITORING

Daily blood glucose monitoring gives you information that is vital to diabetes management. Your child might have an A1C that is acceptable, but if his blood glucose levels are constantly swinging from 50 to 400 mg/dl, that is not optimal blood glucose control. There have been recent indications that swinging blood glucoses over long periods of time cause damage to vessels.

Daily monitoring is done through the use of a blood glucose meter, a small, portable device that checks the glucose levels in your blood. After

Doing the Fingerstick

1. Wash your child's hands with warm, soapy water and dry well.
2. Prepare your meter and test strip according to the manufacturer's instructions.
3. Choose the spot where you are going to do the fingerstick.
4. Place the finger-pricking device on the side of the finger. Press the release mechanism.
5. Squeeze out a drop of blood. If you have a hard time drawing a drop of blood, try this: After sticking the finger, hang the hand down and gently shake it. Lightly squeeze the finger, moving from the middle joint toward the fingertip (this is called "milking" the finger).
6. Place the blood as directed in the instructions for your meter.
7. Wait for the results. Record the number in your daily log.

pricking your skin (typically the side of a finger) with a lancet, you place a tiny drop of blood on a test strip that is inserted into the meter. The meter quickly (usually within 5 seconds) displays the blood glucose level as a number on the meter's digital display. You can compare this number to your target range (see page 10) to see if your glucose level is too high or too low.

If your child has many blood glucose readings outside of the target range, you will need to adjust her insulin, food, or schedule. If you see patterns of high or low blood glucose and are uncertain what to do, call your diabetes educator or diabetes provider for help. Knowing your child's blood glucose level before a meal can help you to decide whether to encourage him to eat an extra helping of food or to give more or less insulin at the next injection. Learning to look for patterns in your child's blood glucose levels will help you to fine-tune his insulin dosages, activity level, and food intake.

If your child is a newborn, your diabetes educator should recommend a blood glucose meter that is approved for use in newborns. Not all meters have been approved for use in newborns.

Since the first blood glucose meters for home use were developed in the 1980's, the technology has grown. They continue to become smaller, lighter, more economical, more efficient, increasingly accurate, and easier to use. User error has also been minimized. They can be conveniently carried in a backpack, purse, or pocket. Your health care provider can teach you how to do blood glucose testing correctly and answer any questions that you may have. In addition, the manufacturers of meters have customer service departments that you can call with questions, concerns, or technical problems.

Tips for Easier, Less Painful Sticks

New pricking devices and fine pointed lancets help to make the stick almost painless. Some of these devices are specially made for children's sensitive fingers. They go deep enough into the skin to draw a small drop of blood but not deep enough to hurt much or leave much of a mark. Ask your diabetes educator or pharmacist to show you these devices.

♦ Prick the sides of the fingers to draw blood. The sides have a good blood supply and fewer nerve endings than the fingertips.

♦ You can also do sticks on the inside of the arm, if your child has not just eaten or exercised. (If she has, the reading may be slightly different than the finger.)

♦ Young children can also be tested in the earlobes, heels, and toes. (In infants, it is safest to use the outer sides of the heels.) It is often hard to capture the drop of blood in a spot such as the earlobe when you have a moving target.

Calloused skin may develop from frequent pricks in one place, and make it even more difficult to get blood out of that spot. Keep rotating the finger prick sites.

Continuous Glucose Monitoring

Recently, technology has moved toward being able to obtain blood glucose levels all the time. Continuous glucose monitoring (CGM) does not replace glucose meters: they work alongside them. A CGM is made up of three parts: a sensor, a transmitter, and a receiver, and records your glucose numbers on a minute-by-minute basis. The CGM measures glucose in your interstitial fluid—the fluid among your cells—rather than your blood. The CGM is useful because it allows you to track high and low trends of your blood glucose levels. It is always reading blood glucose levels and will report them to a pump or other device. This technology is relatively new and can be very helpful to adults and teens to avoid extreme high and low blood glucose. Research has not yet shown it to be greatly effective for use in children but some parents find it very reassuring.

CGM numbers might differ somewhat from meter glucose levels because meters measure capillary blood glucose while CGMs measure serum glucose. Both meters and CGM measure glucose, but differently, so one is not better than the other. The companies that make CGM products advise you to check blood glucose levels with a meter before giving insulin to make sure you are giving yourself the right amount. One of the problems in using CGMs for school-age children or younger is that they are not adept at making changes and do not know what to do with the alerts and alarms when they occur. Some kids get annoyed with the beeping and will shut it off, and others resent having a second site. It takes diligence and some maturity to use it well.

HOW OFTEN TO TEST BLOOD GLUCOSE

Your child's age, eating habits, activity level, and insulin needs, as well as how quickly he is growing and needs to be considered when determining how frequently blood should be tested. The need for continuous glucose monitoring arose from the recognition that our standard therapy was not good enough.

Four blood glucose tests a day (at least) are usually recommended for children and teens. Testing blood glucose levels during the night gives helpful information about how to regulate food and insulin and can help detect nighttime low blood glucose. It is usually recommended that children using multiple daily injections or an insulin pump test at least four times a day and one to two times a week around 3–4 a.m. It is important to do nighttime blood tests if your child has had several low blood glucose levels throughout the day or at bedtime, if she has had an unusually active day, or have not eaten well.

> "Young children are not always able to communicate when they are feeling symptoms. When in doubt—test."

Your doctor may sometimes ask you to test your child's blood glucose levels at other times of day than when you usually do it. This can help you to get a clearer picture of what happens to your child's glucose levels throughout the day.

The more tests that are done, the more information is available to keep blood glucose in the target range. Frequent blood glucose tests are especially important in very young children because they may be unable to communicate if they are feeling symptoms of low or high blood glucose. When in doubt—test! Even children and teens who use continuous monitoring must continue to check blood glucose on a meter when they are taking insulin in case there is a discrepancy in the readings.

Your child's blood glucose may always be normal before meals, but how do you know whether it goes sky high right after meals? The way to find out is to do a test an hour or two after a meal. Continuous glucose monitoring can also be used as a diagnostic tool to learn what is happening between meals and through the night. It is used for exactly this reason. You can use the additional information you get from these tests to help you make decisions about your child's daily food intake and his exercise and insulin routine.

It can also be helpful to check a child's blood glucose after he eats a food that you suspect raises his glucose level significantly. This can help you decide whether to give extra insulin before your child eats that food next time. Extra blood tests when your child is sick can help you decide how to adjust insulin dosages and food. Anytime that your child acts like or says he feels his blood glucose is low, it's a good idea to do a blood test. This can prevent anxious eating—when a child mistakes nervousness for low blood glucose and eats a snack he doesn't need.

Checking blood glucose is helpful before, during, and after exercise. If your child's blood glucose is on the low side before exercise, he should eat or drink an extra 15 grams of carbohydrate. Doing a check during exercise can show you if your child's sweating and pounding heart are caused by exertion or by low blood glucose. (See Playing Games and Sports, page 97.)

Your doctor or diabetes educator will help you to look for patterns in your child's blood glucose readings and decide whether your child's insulin dose needs to be changed.

RECORDING RESULTS OF BLOOD GLUCOSE TESTS

Each time you do a blood glucose test, it's important to record the number as well as the dose of insulin, and anything unusual going on such as illness, special foods, or activity. A log will help you to keep track of this information. By logging this information, you and your diabetes professional can better understand what changes need to be made.

Most meters have a memory that holds a variable number of previous readings. Some meters include the date and time of the test and can be uploaded into a computer program. This is helpful if you forget to record the blood glucose results; however, unless you have a meter that allows you to enter how much insulin is taken, along with other events, it is still important to keep a written record of this information. Your health care provider will probably need the information when making recommendations in your care. It's still best to keep your own records of insulin doses and any special events (sick days, extra exercise, etc.). Otherwise, you may miss patterns and won't be able to determine if changes need to be made. The records are your tools for improving diabetes control. Parents who keep logs such as this make more insulin adjustments than those who don't, which is important to avoid highs and lows.

Look at your records frequently. After uploading your meter into the computer, some people find it helpful to sort their information into graphs and charts. Most computer programs give you the ability to review the data in many different ways, such as such as pie charts, scatter grams, or bar charts. Your written logs have a comments section for recording events during the day, such as exercise, meal times, special treats eaten, low blood glucose symptoms, or illness. These records can help you detect patterns and trends in glucose levels.

HOW TO TEST BLOOD GLUCOSE CORRECTLY

Every brand of meter allows you to check its accuracy so that you know your results are true. One way is to use a "control solution." Control solution tests the accuracy of the system. A drop of the control solution is placed on the test strip and the test strip is read by the meter. The results you get with control solution should be within a certain range, identified on the control solution vial, or package of strips. If you find that your meter is out of the accepted range for accuracy, call the customer service phone number on the back of your meter. The problem might be with the strips or the meter itself. Control solution is made to work with the brand of meter it is sold with, so do not swap brands.

Another way of checking the accuracy of your meter is to compare a sample of blood on your meter with a laboratory result for the blood. If blood is being drawn in a lab for routine blood work, you can check your blood glucose on your meter at the same time. This works best when the same sample of blood is used for both. This way, you can compare the results to see if your meter is reading close to the lab value. Glucose results from capillary blood are about 11% higher than with blood from a vein. If the reading from your meter and the result from the laboratory are within 20% of each other, most diabetes centers consider your meter to be accurate. You should also know whether your meter is scaled to blood serum or whole blood. Serum values are higher.

KETONE TESTING

Ketones are by-products of breaking down body fat. When the body breaks down fat for energy because glucose is not reaching cells, ketones build up. Ketones can cause the blood to become acidic, which leads to nausea, vomiting, and flu-like symptoms. Large amounts of ketones in

Diabetes Weekly Diary

Month: _____ **Year:** _____

Date/Day	Time/Units	Insulin Dose	Blood Glucose and Urine Ketone Test Results									
			Breakfast		Lunch		Dinner		Bedtime		Night	

Reasons for Ketones

Ketones can appear in the urine when your child has:

♦ an illness (blood sugar can be high or low from stress hormones)
♦ not taken enough insulin
♦ emotional stress
♦ not been eating well
♦ recently had an episode of low blood glucose.

the urine can lead to a dangerous condition called ketoacidosis (see page 7). This is a very serious problem that needs careful supervision and treatment. (See warning signs of ketoacidosis, page 9.)

Urine or blood should be tested for the presence of ketones when blood glucose levels are over 250 mg/dl (or 300 depending on your doctor's advice) and especially when your child is sick. Testing for ketones first thing in the morning can alert you to a low blood glucose that might have occurred in the night while your child was asleep.

The least expensive, traditional way to check for ketones is to have your child urinate on a strip that measures ketones. Wait the suggested amount of time, and compare the color to that on the bottle to see if ketones are present in the urine and if so, how large a quantity.

Urine ketones are measured as:

small/trace   +   moderate   ++   large   +++

To get the most accurate readings, follow the manufacturer's instructions for using the test strips. Be sure to keep records of all urine test results. The strips are sensitive to humidity, so don't keep them in the bathroom. It is important to remind your child to recap the bottle immediately after taking a strip out, and also to not use the strips past their expiration date.

Blood ketone testing is more popular and recommended over urine testing. This test is done on a meter with a special strip that reads the presence of ketones in the blood. With blood ketone testing, you can detect the presence of ketones earlier (typically within 10 seconds) than in the urine and begin treatment early, hopefully preventing more serious problems. The meter is also easily portable and convenient when traveling away from home.

When your child is sick, test for ketones every time he urinates or whenever you check blood glucose levels on a meter (every two hours or whatever is recommended by your doctor). Tell your doctor or diabetes educator if you find a large amount of ketones in your child's urine or if ketones are present (even in small amounts) on more than one test.

Ask your doctor for specific information on who to call and what to do when you find ketones in your child's urine. Work with your team to help figure out the reason for the ketones and how to treat them. It is important to offer your child plenty of fluids to help her stay hydrated. You may also need to provide extra insulin until ketones clear.

HELPING YOUR CHILD TEST REGULARLY

Getting your child to do blood glucose testing four or more times a day can be a challenge. Your child may resist testing because he does not feel it is important or doesn't want to get bad news. Sometimes children will say they didn't test because they "knew" they were either high or low. (Research has shown that children and adults cannot accurately guess their blood glucose much of the time.) Others may not want to test because they know that you, their parent, get upset at a high number. Sometimes your child may find it hard to do the testing himself, and you may have to take over for a while.

It might surprise you to learn that falsification of blood glucose numbers is a common problem among children—and adults—with diabetes, and occasionally even parents. Diabetes management is an all-day, everyday, "24/7" burden of responsibility. It's inconvenient for adults and children and having to test four or more times a day is difficult, even with modern technology. It's not surprising that even when children and teens are physically and intellectually capable of carrying out all the tasks of their diabetes self-care, they are not always able to meet the expectations of their health care team and parents.

When records are not accurate, it can be unsafe for the child. The parent or health care team may make changes to insulin doses, food, and exercise to try and fix a problem that doesn't exist. This will throw blood

Common Reasons for Falsifying Numbers

Feeling overwhelmed by the demands of diabetes care or simply not being able to keep up—and not wanting anyone to know about it—are common reasons for children and teens to falsify numbers. Some other reasons that it happens are related to:

♦ The desire to please. ("I want you to be happy with me, so I'll give you what you want to see.")

♦ The desire to avoid your anger. ("Every time my number is high, my dad grills me on what I ate, and what I did, and is mad. It happens even when I didn't do anything wrong, so I think I'll avoid that situation.")

♦ Boundary testing. ("I don't really want to do this. I'll test you to see how much you care whether or not I do this, and see whether it matters!")

♦ Creative exploration for the mere science of it. ("I wonder if I can avoid doing the finger stick and yet make it look real. Could jelly, milk, juice, or hand lotion work instead of blood.")

♦ The desire to be independent. ("I want to do it myself but know I need to make it look good.")

Many children and teens truly want to do it themselves, but are unable to sustain the effort. This is a normal part of child development. The children who do best long term, are those who have parents who stay involved, always checking, always available to supervise, and advise.

glucose further out of target range. One way that parents can encourage honesty in their children is to learn to react less emotionally to blood glucose readings. Parents should be clear about which blood glucose levels require action and what that action should be. They should also be aware of the many factors that can affect blood glucose levels, such as illness or stress. Kids are kids, and will inevitably make mistakes. Some kids do better with monitoring, some with diet, some with injections, some with record keeping, and some with adjustments, but it is extremely rare to find parents and kids who do everything perfectly.

Giving praise each time a test is done or awarding stars or points toward an extra privilege or fun event can help to get your young child to test regularly. Although some parents have been successful with disincentives, such as grounding or loss of cell phone, others feel that having to live with diabetes is enough of a punishment. Positive reinforcement, when applied consistently over a long period of time, is a self-esteem builder. Let your child know that even high numbers give the information needed to control blood glucose. Try not to "freak-out" at the numbers when things are not going well.

Chris thought that doing his blood tests took too much time. He had more homework now that he was in high school. On top of this, he had basketball practices and a part-time job. Chris' parents quizzed him about everything he ate if his glucose reading was high. Chris found that it was easier to just write in some glucose values in his log rather than actually doing the test. Plus, he could write glucose readings that were within his target range and it would get his parents off his case.

When he had his diabetes appointment, the diabetes educator checked his meter's memory and learned that the glucose values didn't match with his logbook. Chris was afraid that his parents and doctor would be angry with him. He was glad that instead of showing disappointment, the doctor and his parents made a deal with him.

The diabetes educator worked with Chris and found out which times of the day he could test without it being a hassle. Chris, his parents, the diabetes educator, and the doctor agreed to a testing schedule that would really work. His parents agreed not to pressure him when he missed a test or if his readings were high. Chris promised to record glucose readings that were real. If Chris successfully worked within the agreement, his parents would allow him to get his driver's permit.

CHAPTER 5:
Nitty-Gritty 3—Meal Plans

Chapter 5:
Nitty-Gritty 3—Meal Plans

Food is a very important part of our lives. Along with the basic need for food for survival, we also use food to celebrate birthdays, holidays, and special events. Certain foods have special meaning for us, like pumpkin pie at Thanksgiving or popcorn at the movies.

Good eating habits have slipped as snack foods, fast foods, and prepared foods have become a common part of our daily lives. Portion sizes have doubled or tripled and soda and sports drinks have replaced milk and water.

Family eating has become a thing of the past, despite the benefits of mealtimes spent together. The social aspects and expectations of having a family meal caused children to learn to respect family time. They learned table manners and to have dinner conversation, and families came together to enjoy each other's company at least once a day. It also opened up the opportunity to eat nutritious, well-balanced meals that were healthy for the entire family. As a parent, you probably have thoughts and concerns about establishing good eating habits—and rightly so. Families who establish good eating habits, have children and teens that eat well and eat healthier foods. And when your child has diabetes, this becomes critically important.

> "Families who establish good eating habits have children and teens who eat well and eat heathier foods."

Your family can continue to enjoy meals—every day and on special occasions. You'll learn new, healthier ways to cook old favorite. You will find that the extra time you spend planning meals will pay off for everyone.

You will learn to pay close attention to what your child eats and when she eats. Food raises blood glucose. Not enough food can cause blood glucose to drop. Planning meals for your child, and/or counting carbohydrates will help balance your child's food, insulin, and exercise.

WHY IS MEAL PLANNING IMPORTANT?

Meal planning for children with diabetes is important for two reasons:

♦ Your child will get the right amount of calories and nutrients to grow and develop normally.

♦ Blood glucose levels will be more easily controlled.

A child's need for nutrients from food depends on age, sex, weight, and activity level. As your child grows, caloric and nutrient needs change. Having a healthy, balanced plan of eating will encourage your child to eat healthy foods and will give some structure to meal preparation.

A general meal plan usually comes from a dietitian when your child is first diagnosed. She will base it on his food preferences and your family patterns of eating. If you see that it is either too much food, or not enough food, you should tell the dietitian so that it can be adjusted. It is your child's meal plan, so it should fit into his life.

Having a dietitian as a member of your health care team is very helpful when it comes to meal planning. The dietitian can answer questions or concerns that you or your child may have. The plan is not hard and fast, but should be able to be changed based on your child's appetite and food choices. It is a guide for healthy eating.

Meal planning for children with diabetes is not handled in the same way as for adults with diabetes. Younger children have small stomachs that hold smaller amounts of food. Kids also need extra calories to grow and develop, so adding snacks becomes very important. Some kids are picky, while other kids will eat anything. Some kids are very active and play sports, while other kids are relatively sedentary. There are all kinds of kids, and their activity levels and eating habits can change constantly, so flexibility is key.

Food-Related Issues

Parents of kids with diabetes think about food-related issues, such as :

♦ how to provide a healthy diet.

♦ how to help my child have a healthy weight.

♦ how to meet dietary needs for one child along with the needs of other family members.

♦ how to promote healthy choices in a child or teen's decision making.

♦ how to handle holidays such as Halloween or birthdays.

♦ how to help one child lose weight and another gain weight.

♦ how to develop eating habits that will promote health for the rest of my child's life.

♦ how to be the best role model for my child.

♦ how to teach my child how to count carbohydrates and balance it with insulin.

Most diabetes centers and dietitians recommend a flexible basal/bolus insulin regimen with carbohydrate counting. This type of regimen is more flexible, so that your child can eat more or less and cover it with an adequate amount of insulin.

LET APPETITE BE YOUR GUIDE

A child's appetite varies widely and usually indicates the need for food. During growth spurts or times of lots of physical activity, your child may eat heartily. Other times, you may wonder how she keeps going on so little food. This is the way children normally eat, and having diabetes doesn't change that. You will learn how to make changes in insulin dose based on your child's appetite. It is also important to make meal times pleasant, which means avoiding a battle of wills over food.

Parts of a Meal Plan

The meal plan is not an absolute guide that can never change, but it is a general plan for a well-balanced diet and good nutrition. It's a good idea to go over your child's eating habits and meal plan once a year with your dietitian to make sure it is still right for them. Even though you might be counting carbohydrates in order to balance insulin, the plan will give you an idea of:

♦ an appropriate amount of food for your child.

♦ the amounts of fruits and vegetables to include.

♦ the timing of meals and snacks.

♦ a plan for how much fat, cholesterol, and sugar your child should eat.

♦ how to regulate food and insulin. (This balance means matching insulin doses to the amount of food eaten.)

When your child was diagnosed with diabetes, she may have lost weight or perhaps not gained weight for a while. Once treatment begins, she may have a tremendous appetite and eat well. After the weight is gained she may not want so much food. Your dietitian will give you guidelines at diagnosis, but you may need to increase or decrease the number of calories to keep up with her appetite. Therefore, you'll need to keep in touch with your dietitian when making meal plan changes and deciding how much insulin to give to balance the food.

If she's hungry, you can give your child extra food, but do it at mealtimes when it can be covered with insulin. Give your child seconds on foods from all the food groups, not just extra potatoes or bread. On the other hand, if she does not eat well at a meal, try giving her milk or juice to help keep her blood glucose level up until the next meal. Your diabetes educator or dietitian will be able to tell you how to adjust insulin according to what your child eats. Adjusting insulin to food works best if you are following a carbohydrate counting plan (see page 83).

The Big Three

The three major nutrients our bodies get from all foods are carbo-hydrates, protein, and fat. These nutrients do different things in the body.

Carbohydrates are the body's main source of energy. They are found in fruits, vegetables, bread, cereal, milk, rice, potatoes, and pasta. These foods are turned into glucose during digestion easily, which increases the blood glucose level fairly quickly.

Protein is used to build and repair body tissue. It is found in meat, poultry, fish, eggs, cheese, peanut butter, tofu, and milk.

Fat provides reserves of energy. It is found in marbled meat, the skin of poultry, whole milk, butter, cheese, and oils such as corn oil and olive oil. It is difficult for the body to turn fat into glucose. Fat has little effect on the blood glucose level other than slowing down digestion and absorption of carbohydrate.

A BALANCED DIET

Children should eat a well-balanced diet that includes fruits and vegetables and is low in fat and high in fiber. Children with diabetes are no exception. These days you can pretty much eat what you were eating before you got diabetes. BUT, and this is an important BUT, you have to plan before you eat. The intention of planning meals is to control eating so that your child has a program of well-balanced nutrition, a healthy amount of calories, and a way of balancing insulin to food. There are a number of approaches to meal planning and sometimes you might combine a couple of them after seeing what works best for your family.

All food is organized into groups based on what it is made of, and how the body uses it. These groups are generally, grains and breads, milk and dairy products, fruits and vegetables, meat and meat substitutes, and fats and sweets. If your child eats a wide variety of foods from each of the food groups, vitamin and mineral supplements are usually not necessary.

Carbohydrates and Sugars

Glucose is the body's main energy source. Glucose is released from the liver and also comes from foods that we eat, mostly from carbohydrates. Before it can be used as energy, glucose must get inside the body's cells.

Carbohydrates are found in fruits, vegetables, bread, cereal, milk, rice, potatoes, pasta, chips, sweets, and sugary beverages. Foods like bread, potatoes, and pasta are called starches or complex carbohydrates. The body breaks them down into glucose.

sugar

Sugar (sucrose) is a carbohydrate. For many years, health professionals thought that people with diabetes should avoid foods that contain sugar. We now know that foods that contain sugar, when eaten as part of a meal, have about the same effect on blood glucose levels as other carbohydrates. For example, a dessert brownie that has 15 grams of carbohydrate will affect your child's blood glucose level about the same as a potato with margarine, which also has about 15 grams of carbohydrate. This means that foods containing sugar can be part of your child's meal plan as long as:

♦ they are eaten in small amounts
♦ your child's blood glucose levels are checked regularly
♦ you monitor the total amount of carbohydrate in your child's diet and adjust insulin accordingly.

It's a good idea to encourage your child to eat only a small amount of sugary foods. Most of these foods have little nutritional value and they are often high in fat. Talk to your dietitian about the best way to fit some sweet treats into your child's meal plan.

fruit and fruit juice

Fruit and fruit juice contain natural sugar (fructose) and other important nutrients. Your dietitian will recommend how much fruit your child with diabetes should eat at each meal or snack.

Sugary foods and juice are usually more concentrated in carbohydrate in a small serving, so portion size is key when carb counting. When your child has low blood glucose, the first step is to give him a food high in carbohydrate, such as a glucose tablet, regular soda, or juice. Follow it up with crackers or a sandwich if it is going to be a long time until the next meal or snack.

At certain times you may want to give your child a snack that might contain fruit juice or a sugar in order to raise her blood glucose. The following are examples of times when you may want to do this:

♦ to balance a low blood glucose reading
♦ during or after exercise if blood sugar is dropping
♦ during a long gap between meals if blood sugar is under 80 mg/dl
♦ on sick days if blood glucose is low

fat and cholesterol

Unless your child is younger than 2, her meal plan should limit the amount of fat and cholesterol that she eats. The U.S. government's healthy eating guidelines advise all Americans over age 2 to eat less fat (especially saturated fat) and cholesterol to reduce the chances of getting heart disease.

Saturated fat and cholesterol are found mostly in animal products, including butter, lard, whole milk, and fatty meats. Using low-fat milk and cheese and eating lean meat will help you and your child to eat less saturated fat.

Fat and Cholesterol Recommendations

For any child or adolescent (2 to 18 years of age), the following pattern of nutrient intake is recommended:

1. saturated fatty acids < 10% of total calories;
2. total fat over several days of < 30% of total calories and no less than 20% of total calories;
3. dietary cholesterol < 300 mg per day.

American Academy of Pediatrics Guidelines: Pediatrics, 101 (1), January 1998, pp 141–147.

HOW DO I PLAN MEALS?

Meal plans generally include three meals and two or three snacks a day depending on your child's age and schedule. Young children typically eat smaller quantities of food but need food more frequently. Older kids can go longer periods of time without eating. It is a good idea for your child to eat at about the same time of day whenever possible.

Your child's schedule won't be exactly the same every day. It's okay to adjust your child's meal plan when your family's schedule changes. When you know that a meal is going to be eaten later than usual, make sure a snack is available or eaten to keep her blood glucose from getting too low. If your child is using a basal/bolus plan with a long-acting insulin or pump, it is less of an issue because typically she will not take bolus insulin until she is ready to eat.

Because most children have normal blood pressure and cholesterol levels, a low-sodium, low fat, high fiber diet plan is not a crucial component of the meal plan. On the other hand, preventing high blood pressure and obesity is important. The dietary plan should reflect a generally well-balanced healthy eating plan and be modified if there are concerns about weight or blood pressure. It is well known that people with diabetes are more prone to heart disease and high blood pressure, so although it is not essential to restrict fat and sodium in children and teens, it makes sense to be prudent about it. Eating less unhealthy (saturated and trans) fat and sodium can help reduce the risk of developing these problems. Healthy eating guidelines developed by the U.S. government advise Americans to cut the fat in their diets to no more than 30% of all calories they eat. Your dietitian or other health care provider can help you to plan meals that are both healthy and enjoyable. Some examples of meal planning options are below.

Meal Planning and Portion Control

A meal plan is basically giving your child a well-balanced diet suitable for his age and weight, and is based on portion sizes. One widely used method of meal planning is *Choose Your Foods: Exchange Lists for Diabetes* (American Diabetes Association, 2008). This meal plan has foods grouped according to similar nutrition content and serving sizes. One serving is known as an exchange or choice.

When meal planning, foods are divided into six categories based on the amount of carbohydrate, protein, and fat they contain. Each serving of the food has about the same amount of carbohydrate, protein, fat, and calories as other foods on the same list. Try to spread your meals throughout the day and do not skip meals. The categories are: starch, vegetables, fruits, milk and yogurt, meat and meat substitutes, and fats.

Young children will often be started on this type of meal plan so that meals can be as consistent as possible. Your child's individual meal plan tells you how many portions can be chosen from each list at a meal. The goal is to make sure that your child eats the right amount of nutrients each day.

Sample Foods for Each Exchange List

♦ Starch: bread, hot and dry cereal, rice, pasta, and crackers. It also contains starchy vegetables: potatoes, corn, peas, and beans.

♦ Vegetables: all fresh, frozen, and canned vegetables and vegetable juices (all nonstarchy vegetables).

♦ Fruits: all fresh, frozen, canned, and dried fruit or fruit juices.

♦ Milk and Yogurt: Fat-free and low-fat milk and yogurt are the healthiest choices. (Cream cheese, cream, and butter are found in the fats group, while cheese is in the meat and meat substitutes.)

♦ Meat and Meat Substitutes: meats, poultry, seafood, eggs, cheese, and peanut butter. (These foods provide you with much of the protein you need.)

♦ Fats: oils, butter, margarine, salad dressing, nuts, bacon, and any other fats and oils you use to prepare food.

Planning Meals Using Portion Sizes

The following are examples of meals you might plan for your child using portion control. (2,200-calorie plan)

Breakfast: 1 milk, 1 fruit, 2 starches, and 2 meats
1 cup (8 oz) fat-free (skim) milk (1 milk)
half-cup (4 oz) orange juice (1 fruit)
2 slices of bread (2 starches)
2 slices of lean ham (2 meats)

Lunch: 3 starches, 2 meats, 1 fruit, 1 milk, and 3 fats
grilled cheese sandwich (2 starches, 2 meats, 1 fat)
small apple (1 fruit)
1 cup (8 oz) fat-free (skim) milk (1 milk)
1 oz pretzels (1 starch)

Afternoon snack: 1 starch, 1 milk
3 cups air-popped popcorn (1 starch)
1 cup (8 oz) fat-free yogurt (1 milk)

Dinner: 3 starches, 3 meats, 1 fruit, 1 milk, 2 fats,
        and 2 vegetables
salad with 1 Tbsp dressing (1 vegetable, 1 fat)
medium potato (1 starch)
3 oz baked chicken (3 meats)
2-inch roll (1 starch)
green beans (1 vegetable)
baked apple (1 fruit)
1 cup (8 oz) fat-free (skim) milk (1 milk)

Bedtime snack: 1 starch, 1 meat, and 1 milk
1/2 turkey sandwich (1 starch, 1 meat)
1 cup (8 oz) fat-free (skim) milk (1 milk)

Carbohydrate Counting

Another approach to meal planning is to count the number of carbohydrates in the food consumed. A dietitian will give you guidance about how much carbohydrate to include for meals and snacks. By counting how many carbohydrates are consumed, you can determine how much insulin to give. This approach makes things more flexible as your child can eat more or less as long as you adjust the insulin accordingly.

Your provider, educator, or dietitian will give you a number, based on the weight, age, development, and insulin sensitivity of your child, called your child's "carb ratio." Basically, it is the number of grams of carbohydrate covered by 1 unit of insulin. For example, 7-year-old Camille has a carb ratio of 1 unit of insulin to 23 grams of carb. On the other hand, 14-year-old Thomas has a carb ratio of 12. Before they eat, they or their parent adds up how much carbohydrate they plan to eat and divides that total by 23 or 12, respectively. So, if they are both eating 48 g of carb at a meal, Camille will get roughly 2 units to cover it, and Thomas will get 4 units.

Then, added to the dose to cover carbs, is another amount usually called the "correction" or "insulin sensitivity factor." This is an amount of insulin that will correct a high blood sugar, and bring it down into a target goal range. So, in Camille's case, her doctor figured out that her correction is "75" or in other words, 1 unit of insulin will drop her blood glucoses about 75 mg/dl. Her target goal is to be 100 mg/dl, so if she checks her blood glucose and it is 175 mg/dl, it would take 1 unit to bring her back into goal. (Blood glucose minus 100 mg/dl) divided by 75 = 1 unit.

In Thomas's case, because he is in the middle of a growth spurt and puberty, his doctor suggests a correction of 25. His formula would be (Blood glucose minus 100 mg/dl) divided by 25, which if his blood glucose was 175 mg/dl to start, would be 3 units. So, the amount to cover the food and the amount to correct the blood glucose are added together. Insulin pumps do this for you, and as long as you have correct parameters programmed into the pump and do a good job accurately measuring the carbs, the pump should give you a very precise amount of insulin.

Pumps also know how much insulin your child has taken and will subtract that amount from the suggested total dose. So, to eat the same amount of carbs with similar blood sugars, Camille's formula would give her 3 total units, and Thomas's formula would give him 7 units. This system only works well, however, if you and your child can be very consistent about reading labels, portion sizes, and weighing or measuring the food.

Estimated Insulin to Carbohydrate Ratio

The following is a rough estimate of how many grams of carbohydrate one unit of insulin will cover in a child based on weight. Differences may occur, however, if you child is recently diagnosed, is in the middle of puberty, or has insulin resistance.

Weight in Pounds	Grams of Carbs
50–59	31
60–69	28
70–79	25
80–99	22
90–99	19
110–109	16
110–129	15
130–139	14
140–149	13
150–159	12
160–169	11
170–179	10
180–189	9
190–199	8

The Plate Method

The plate method is another meal planning method of controlling portions and healthy eating. This method is particularly helpful when food portions are difficult to determine, like when eating at a restaurant. The idea behind the plate method is pretty simple: fill half of the plate with non-starchy vegetables, one quarter should be filled with lean protein, and the other quarter should contain carbohydrates. You can also include a cup of milk and fruit. For breakfast, it is a little difficult but is the same general format. Half of your plate contains carbohydrates and one quarter may contain protein (this is optional). It also includes a cup of milk and one piece of fruit.

Although the plate method is easy in theory, difficulty can arise if your child is a picky eater or they will not eat fruits and vegetables (which unfortunately is true of many kids).

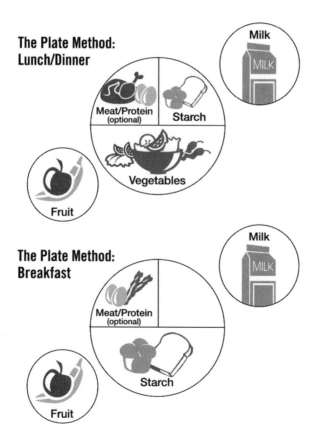

Alternative Sweeteners

Alternative sweeteners are products that can be used instead of sugar to sweeten food. People with and without diabetes can safely use alternative sweeteners. Most (but not all) alternative sweeteners have few calories. Most dietitians suggest the use of artificial sweeteners for children with diabetes in moderation. There has been no consensus about what "moderation" means in a child's diet. A general guideline, based on the age of your child, might be to limit diet drinks to two per day in children over 10 years old and one per day in children under 10. There are six artificial sweeteners currently approved by the US Food and Drug Administration (FDA). Other natural substitutes are known, but are yet to gain official approval for food use.

non-nutritive sweeteners

The FDA regulates artificial sweeteners as food additives. Saccharin is about 400 times as sweet as sugar. People with diabetes can safely use saccharin. A possible disadvantage of saccharin is that it can leave a slightly bitter aftertaste.

Aspartame is about 200 times as sweet as sugar. Most people, including people with diabetes, can safely use aspartame. Aspartame is not safe for people who have a rare condition called phenylketonuria (PKU). Aspartame can't be used for cooking in recipes that require lengthy heating or cooking. Use in recipes that have been tested.

Sucralose, a sugar deritive, has no calories. It is a good choice for cooking or baking, as well as to sprinkle on cereal, fruit, or anything else.

Neotame is not yet widely used in our foods but was approved by the FDA in 2003. It is made by NutraSweet and is 7,000–13,000 times sweeter than sugar. Although it is structurally related to aspartame, it is dangerous for people born with PKU.

Acesulfame-K contains natural flavors extracted from fruits. It can be used safely by people with diabetes or PKU.

Stevia (rebaudiana) comes from a plant in the sunflower family and has an intense sweetening quality. It is up to 300 times sweeter than sugar, and has no calories. It has been widely used in other countries, such as Japan, and is now catching on in the U.S.

nutritive sweeteners

Fructose (fruit sugar) is naturally found in fruit, so it is not calorie-free like other artificial sweeteners. It is a carbohydrate that is broken down by the body more slowly than other sugars. Fructose should be counted for its carbohydrate contribution in a meal plan for diabetes.

Some non-sugar sweeteners are known as "sugar alcohols." These are, in general, less sweet than sucrose, but have similar bulk properties and can be used in a wide range of food products. Examples of sugar alcohols are mannitol, sorbitol, and xylitol (all ending in "ol"). These sugar alcohols are often found in foods that are labeled "sugar-free" (sugar-free chocolate or sugar-free cookies). They have more slowly absorbed carbohydrate properties and can cause diarrhea. Pediatric dietitians will often suggest that they would prefer a child to eat a piece of regular chocolate or cookie rather than the sugar-alcohol variety as long as the carbohydrates are counted. This is because carbohydrate absorption is more predictable and there is no risk of diarrhea.

BECOMING A FOOD DETECTIVE

Different foods affect people in various ways. There are differences in how quickly foods are used by the body. You may begin to notice that some foods affect your child's blood glucose level more than others. For example, a spaghetti dinner may make her blood glucose run higher than eating mashed potatoes and meat loaf. Waffles for breakfast may cause a rise in blood glucose before lunch, but cereal may not. Pizza prepared at different places may have different effects on blood glucose. Some carbohydrates take longer to convert into glucose while others take less time.

Some foods with an equal amount of carbs can cause a faster or higher rise in blood glucose than other. All carbohydrates behave differently in our bodies. This is called the "glycemic index" (GI) of foods. The GI describes this difference by ranking carbohydrates according to their effect on our blood glucose levels. Choosing low GI carbs—the ones that produce only small fluctuations in our blood glucose and insulin levels—is one secret to stable blood glucose levels.

For example, potatoes have a high glycemic index. This does not mean that your child should not eat potatoes. Potatoes are a healthy food, but you might expect higher blood sugar after a nice serving of mashed potatoes. If you know this information ahead of time, you can adjust insulin accordingly. www.glycemicindex.com has a database so you can check the glycemic index and carbohydrate content of your favorite foods.

As you become aware of the effects that different foods have, you can use this knowledge to balance these foods with insulin or exercise. For example, if you know that a certain type of crackers make your child's blood glucose run higher than pretzels, you may want to pack those crackers for her snack on a day when she is going skating. If waffles make her blood glucose run high, you know that your child will need extra insulin on waffle days.

Keeping a daily log of what your child eats can help you identify how different foods affect your child's blood glucose. You can use this food diary to adjust your child's insulin dosage depending on what she is eating. This sort of detective work takes time and effort. The reward is that you and your child can have more control over her diabetes. Your diabetes educator can help you become skilled at this kind of analysis.

HELP YOUR CHILD ACCEPT A MEAL PLAN

Even though your child's meal plan can be flexible enough to work in a favorite food or dessert, there may be times when you don't want your child to eat what everyone else is eating, so she can have better blood glucose control. These decisions can be difficult, because as a parent you want your child to feel part of the group and not be singled out as being different. However, just like children who have food allergies, there are times when it is not in your child's best interest to eat a particular food.

One of the best approaches is to stay positive and flexible about food choices, while realizing that there will be times when you must say "No" to your child. There may be other times where you allow the food choice with the understanding that her blood glucose might have to run high for a period of time. And other times, your child might accept a favorite healthy substitute without complaining.

Your child's health and safety is a primary concern, but diabetes is a lifelong condition, and feeling deprived or set apart from his friends can cause long-term resistance to diabetes management.

Each situation that comes up may be different, and you will need to have the skills and understanding to make decisions along the way. How you decide to do this depends on the situation, the timing of the food, whether you are able to make an adjustment in insulin easily, your child's frame of mind about the food or situation, and her blood glucose level.

Try to include your child in the decision. If your child's blood glucose level is running high and she really doesn't care that much for the chocolate cake being served, you may decide together to go with the usual meal plan that day and skip the cake. Or, if she feels strongly about eating the cake, you may work out a compromise.

> "The best approach is to figure out a way that your child can have what he wants and still keep his blood glucose levels in his range."

As your child grows and learns about diabetes, it will be important that she understands about food groups and carbohydrates and how they affect her blood glucose levels. Learning this will take time and patience, but it will allow her to make her own decisions about when to choose pretzels over a cupcake, or how to adjust if she eats the cupcake.

It is helpful if everyone in the family eats the same meal instead of serving a separate meal for the child with diabetes. That way, there's no reason for the child with diabetes to feel different. Besides, a meal that is healthy for a person with diabetes is healthy for everyone.

Sometimes your child can have food that looks a lot like the food others are eating. For example, when her friends are having hamburgers, potato chips, and cola, your child can have a broiled hamburger, baked potato chips, and a diet soda. Your child's food is similar to her friends' food, but it is lower in fat and sugar.

With a bit of planning, your child can have lunch at school with her friends. Many schools give out copies of lunch menus for parents who

Seven-year-old Amy's blood test results were often high when she came home from school. Her parents suspected she was eating extra treats on the school bus. Her mother put Amy on her lap, hugged her, and asked her if she was eating candy with her friends. Amy admitted that she was. She said she wanted to join in with what her friends were doing. Amy and her mother talked about how hard it was for her not to eat candy when her friends were eating it. Her mother explained that eating too many candies made Amy's glucose high and that high glucose made Amy feel thirsty and tired. Amy and her parents talked it out and came to an agreement; Amy can have candy on the bus twice a week, as long as mom knows so that she can adjust her insulin, so she won't feel left out. Engaging your children in the solution can make everyone happy.

need to plan their children's meals ahead of time. Use these menus to help your child choose foods that fit in with her meal plan.

Involving your child in planning meals and snacks is always smart. She may find it easier to follow a meal plan that she has helped to influence.

Some children may go through a phase of hiding candy in their school locker or having a cookie and ice cream binge after school. Your child may be rebelling at feeling different, or may be testing you to see what will happen if she eats whatever she wants.

Try to maintain open communication with her if she's having difficulty. Maintain your composure rather than becoming upset or punitive. It will help your child trust that she can share this information with you. Sensitive children might not want to worry you.

Ask her to let you know if or when she snacks on sweets. This information will help you to adjust her insulin. Having a meal plan that is flexible and includes some sweets may prevent your child from bingeing or sneaking food. Praise her with positive reinforcement when she follows her meal plan.

Children feel invisible throughout their early years and teenage years, so dwelling on long-term complications is not usually effective and can be frightening. Talk to your kids and make sure they feel included in decisions. Find out what is important to them and work that into the conversation. For example, if your child loves football and wants to be able to play, explain his diabetes to him in terms of how he might perform for football practice and games. He wants to do his best, so explain to him how caring for his diabetes will make him perform well and feel great on the football field.

COPING WITH SCHEDULE CHANGES

A schedule change will sometimes prevent your child from following her usual meal plan. If sticking to the meal plan means singling her out and upsetting her, it may be better to adjust the meal plan for the schedule change. However, your child's diabetes control may not be the best on these occasions. Changes are easier with basal/bolus insulin.

A special event at school may mean that the time of your child's lunch hour or gym class is changed for a few days. If you know about this change ahead of time, you can add a snack to the meal plan or adjust the insulin dose to maintain balance. It can help to talk with your child's teachers and ask them to inform you whenever there is a change to the school schedule that affects your child's meal times or exercise routine, so you can plan ahead. You might need to adjust insulin around an activity or field trip. If your child uses an insulin pump, you might consider using a temporary basal rate for the day. (See Communicating with Your Child's School, page 144.)

Keeps Snacks On Hand

If lunch is delayed for more than an hour for some reason, it is smart to give your child a snack that contains about 15 grams of carbohydrate (such as 6 low-fat crackers, 2 pretzels, or 3 graham crackers) to keep in the classroom in order to prevent low blood glucose. Additional snacks are helpful anytime your child gets extra exercise or has to wait longer than usual between meals.

HOLIDAYS AND PARTIES

Holidays are extra-special times for children, and eating is often a central part of holiday celebrations. Having diabetes doesn't have to prevent your child from enjoying these special occasions. With careful planning, she can eat most of the same foods that everyone else is eating.

Try to limit the food extravagances to the actual day of the holiday instead of the whole holiday season. Arrange other types of treats, like small toys or extra privileges, for each day of the season.

Plan ahead so that extra foods, such as Grandma's special pie, baked goods, and candy, can be covered with extra insulin. Otherwise, help your child to stick to her meal plan. Try some of the following hints to help your child focus on the festivities instead of the food.

The holiday dinner is not usually a problem, although extra insulin may be needed. However, in some families, the meal falls in mid-afternoon. There are several ways to approach an unusual schedule, so it is important to talk to your diabetes educator to decide the best way to cover the meal with insulin. Harder to deal with are the sweets and

Tips for Holidays and Parties

Easter

♦ Fill an Easter basket with treats other than food, such as coloring books, stickers, clothing, or jewelry.

♦ Fill plastic eggs with promises of treats, like a chance to stay up late or a trip to a museum or to the movies.

Halloween

♦ Have your child trade that trick-or-treat bag full of sweets for a present she has been wanting.

♦ Let them trick-or-treat with their friends and discuss how to work some candy into their plan. This will allow them to feel like a normal kid, while not gorging themselves on candy.

♦ Take a trip to visit a haunted house or see a scary movie.

goodies that may be available for days on end. Talk to your child about having one treat she really likes with her meal, and balance her insulin and exercise accordingly. Keep tempting treats out of reach during the day.

The excitement of holidays can affect children's blood glucose levels. For example, the thrill of opening presents on Christmas morning can distract a child from eating and cause low blood glucose. You can adjust for this by reducing insulin or reminding your child to eat.

When your child does eat sweets, try to problem-solve how much insulin it takes to cover the extra food. Figure out how many grams of carbohydrate are in the food, have your child test her blood glucose, giving her a certain amount of insulin, have her eat the food, then test again 2 hours later. Your doctor, nurse, or dietitian can help with this. Usually, 15 grams of carbohydrate is the equivalent of about 1 unit of insulin for older kids and adults. Teens may need a lower carb ratio, meaning more insulin.

Many party foods are sweet and high in fat. If your child is going to a party, you may want to get in touch with the hosts beforehand to find out what kind of food is being served. If a lot of high-fat, high-sugar foods are on the menu, you may want to offer to bring some healthier choices. For example, popcorn or cereal snacks can substitute for candy at a child's birthday party. Most parents will welcome the offer.

Ashleigh eats dinner at 5 p.m. and plans to go to a party from 6–8 p.m. The party theme is a tea party, with very little activity planned. Ashleigh wants to eat the birthday cake, yet cake and icing always make her glucose levels high. Ashleigh had a rapid-acting insulin before dinner, but ate less than usual. Her mother gave her an extra 1 1/2 units after she arrived at the party to cover the cake she was going to eat. Her mom also spoke to the host parents to let them know that she had insulin to cover the cake and was allowed to eat it. Ashleigh was part of the group, enjoyed the birthday cake, and still prevented her glucose levels from going too high.

It's okay for your child to eat birthday cake or other party foods. It's worth some planning ahead to help keep your child from feeling left out. Before your child goes to a party, it's smart to make plans with her about how she wants to eat and why.

Adjust insulin or alter the amount of food at other meals or the timing of meals to account for the party foods. Sometimes the extra food is substituted for a snack or for part of a meal. At other times, it's eaten in addition to the child's usual food. Plan a calorie-burning family outing after the party.

Your diabetes educator can help you to plan for special events. The box below provides some ideas for children's parties that your child with diabetes can enjoy.

Party Ideas for Children with Diabetes

A picnic or entertainment where kids can be active, have fun, and eat pizza is more in line with today's birthday celebrations. The following are suggestions for parties for kids with diabetes.

♦ Have a soft-dough pretzel-making party. Children enjoy molding the dough into different shapes and then eating their creations as snacks.

♦ Have an apple party. Children might dunk for apples; decorate apple-people with raisins, toothpicks, and grapes; and enjoy an apple dessert.

♦ Have a Mexican fiesta. Children can put together their own tacos.

♦ Have a Hawaiian luau. You can serve pineapple and chicken and the children can wear grass skirts and leis.

♦ Take children swimming or on an outing to the zoo. Your library can be a good source of ideas for children's activities that focus on something other than food.

♦ Put candles on a pizza instead of on a cake.

EATING OUT

Like other special occasions involving food, eating out can be safe and enjoyable for people with diabetes. Many restaurants and fast food chains provide information on the calorie and fat content of menu items. Some offer exchange lists to make meal planning easier. Ask questions about things on the menu. Most restaurant staff will be happy to answer your questions.

If you can't find out the nutritional information at the restaurant, there are various resources you can use to find out the nutritional content. Websites like calorieking.com, dietfacts.com, and dwlz.com all have extensive nutritional information for a variety of restaurants. Along with websites, there are a number of books published that list complete nutritional information for chain and fast-food restaurants. The American Diabetes Association publishes *Guide To Healthy Restaurant Eating*, *Guide to Healthy Fast-Food Eating*, and *The Diabetes Carbohydrate and Fat Gram Guide*. Calorie King publishes *The Calorie King Calorie, Fat, and Carbohydrate Counter 2011*.

Eating away from home means food won't always show up when you expect it. If your meal is taking longer to appear on the table than you planned and you're worried about your child's blood glucose dropping low, ask for some rolls, crackers, or juice. If you're at an event where you're not sure when food will be served, such as a wedding reception, wait to inject insulin until you know that food is within reach.

Helpful Hints for Eating Out

- ♦ Ask if food is breaded or fried before ordering it.
- ♦ Request that meats be broiled rather than fried.
- ♦ Ask if sauces are sweetened.
- ♦ Request that dishes be served without butter, fats, or oils.
- ♦ Ask that salad dressings, margarine, sour cream, and sauces be served on the side.
- ♦ Ask for lite or sugar-free syrup, jelly, or dressing.

CHAPTER 6:
Playing Sports and Games

Chapter 6:
Playing Sports and Games

When children first develop diabetes they may wonder, "Can I still play with my friends or go out for sports?" The answer is YES! Reassure your child that professional athletes with diabetes have played in all the national leagues.

All children should be encouraged to be physically active, and children with diabetes are no exception. Regular exercise has many benefits:

◆ It strengthens the heart and lungs.
◆ It builds muscle and improves flexibility in the joints.
◆ It builds confidence and reduces stress.
◆ It provides interaction with other children.
◆ It helps with weight control.

When the body's muscles are working, more glucose moves into muscle tissue instead of staying in the blood. Children who exercise regularly usually need less insulin than other kids do. This is true for all kids—with or without diabetes. The more physcially fit they are, the better insulin is utilized. Taking part in gym class and team sports also helps your child to develop social skills, and make friends.

For people with diabetes physical activity has an added benefit: it helps to lower blood glucose levels. Although exercise has not been shown to make blood glucose control easier, it is still an important and necessary part of treating diabetes. Because it is difficult to estimate how much food is required to cover a certain amount of exercise, children who exercise strenuously often find that blood glucose numbers vary considerably. It is important to learn how to manage the effect of exercise by doing frequent monitoring of blood glucose. (Be sure to consult with your health care provider before initiating any change in your child's insulin dose.)

Fun Ways To Add Exercise Into Your Day

There are lots of ways to get exercise. It doesn't always mean you have to go out and run several miles, join a gym, or play on a sports team. The only requirement is that your child moves her body and enjoys what she is doing. Make it fun!

♦ Dancing

♦ Biking

♦ Martial arts

♦ Kickball

♦ Swimming

♦ Skateboarding

♦ Baseball, Football, Basketball, Soccer, Hockey

Getting exercise regularly is important for people with diabetes because of the need to balance the effect of exercise with food and insulin. Activities that meet often, at specific times of day, for a specific length of time, make it easier to plan meals and insulin doses. For example, if your child has soccer practice every Monday, Wednesday, and Friday night from 4–6 p.m., it is much easier to plan meals and insulin doses than if the time or days change from week to week.

This chapter provides general guidance on making physical activity and exercise as safe as possible for children with diabetes. If you have specific questions about what's right for your child, check with your doctor or diabetes educator.

BEING PREPARED FOR UNPLANNED ACTIVITIES

Your health care provider can help you to make regular, planned exercise an enjoyable and safe part of your child's life. But children's lives often involve a lot of unplanned activity. For example, your child may take part in a spontaneous basketball game or some other strenuous activity with friends. Because exercise lowers blood glucose levels, unplanned physical activity may cause your child's blood glucose to drop. The simplest way to prevent this is to have him carry glucose tablets or another fast-acting carbohydrate to prevent or treat low blood glucose levels. It's a good idea for your child to eat a snack before taking part in any unplanned strenuous physical activity, especially if your child is not using an insulin pump. (On a pump, he can turn down the rate of delivery.)

Depending on how strenuous the activity is, additional snacks may be needed during the play or afterward. These snacks are eaten in addition to the child's usual meals. They replace the glucose that the muscle cells use during exercise. How much food your child needs to eat depends on what his blood glucose level is and how strenuous the activity is. By checking blood glucose levels before the activity, you and your child can decide how much extra food is needed.

Guidelines for Snacks and Exercise

The following are general guidelines for snacks before exercise. A dietitian may suggest other guidelines for your child. Consult your health care provider for specific advice.

Light activities (such as walking, bowling, or ping-pong)

♦ Carbohydrate need: 20–30 grams per hour of exercise

♦ Blood glucose 70–180 mg/dl: 3–5 pretzels or 2–3 cups of popcorn would provide 10–15 grams of carbohydrate

♦ Blood glucose over 180 mg/dl: A snack may not be required before light exercise, or it can be eaten after the exercise.

Vigorous activities (such as jogging or competitive swimming)

♦ Carbohydrate need: 30–60 grams per hour of exercise

♦ Blood glucose 70–180 mg/dl: 1–2 sandwiches or 1 sandwich and 1 piece of fruit eaten before exercise provides enough complex carbohydrate and protein for 1 hour of strenuous exercise.

♦ Blood glucose above 180 mg/dl: 1 sandwich or 1 fruit

HOW TO MAKE SURE YOUR CHILD PLAYS SAFELY

As well as carrying snack foods like crackers or pretzels, it's a good idea for youngsters to carry a backup source of glucose to guard against lows. Always keep some form of sugar, hard candy, or glucose tablets in your child's backpack, purse, or pocket.

Talk with your child's gym teachers and sports coaches about the symptoms of low blood glucose and what to do if it occurs (see page 107). It's important that your child exercise with a buddy whenever possible in case he has an episode of low blood glucose and needs help. Make sure the buddy knows what to do or how to get help.

> " It's important that your child exercise with a buddy whenever possible in case he has an episode of low blood glucose. "

Lengthy exercise (like a day-long ski trip) or a major change in routine (like the start of football training) requires special planning. Talk to your health care provider about how to prepare for these kinds of activities.

Strenuous exercise like jogging or swimming laps can affect glucose levels up to 24 hours later. Even if your child snacks before strenuous exercise, he may still have low blood glucose afterward. It's generally suggested that blood glucose be checked during the night on a day when the child has had more exercise than usual.

Many sports teams are now providing drinks and snacks. Sometimes the snacks come from parents, and sometimes the school or coach has them available. As a parent, ask what is being consumed by your child while at practice. Sometimes your child may be drinking too much of a sports drink that contains carbs, or eating oranges, or other snacks provided. It will be important to know what is served, and what your child would like to eat, before making a decision about what to do. You might need to talk to coaches, your child, and your diabetes educator or dietitian for ideas on how to allow your child to fully participate, yet keep blood sugar levels from dropping or skyrocketing.

BALANCING EXERCISE AND INSULIN

What if you take all these precautions and your child still has lows during gym class or while playing games? If that happens, your child's insulin dosage may need to be decreased.

Insulin will likely need to be decreased if your child is taking part in a vigorous sport like swimming, soccer, or football, and doesn't want to load up on food beforehand. Big changes in your child's insulin dosage should only be made after discussion with your doctor. You can, however, learn how to fine-tune your child's dosage to control glucose levels. (See Adjusting Insulin at Home, page 40.)

Children should not exercise if ketones are present in their urine. Exercise causes fat to be broken down and can increase the amount of ketones in the body. (See Ketone Testing, page 64.) Ketones can be a sign that there is too little insulin available.

Precautions for Safe Physical Activity

Before exercise

♦ Check blood glucose level.
♦ Eat an extra carbohydrate-rich snack and/or take less insulin.

At all times

♦ Carry glucose tablets to treat lows.
♦ Don't exercise if ketones are present in the blood or urine.
♦ During strenuous exercise, stop every 30 minutes to eat or drink a carbohydrate-rich snack.
♦ Tell your teammates, coach, or person you're exercising with the signs to look for in case you start to go low. Also teach them what to do to help you.
♦ Always wear your medical ID bracelet.

After exercise

♦ Check your blood glucose often after exercising. The effects of exercise on your blood glucose can last for up to 30 hours.

CHAPTER 7:
Highs and Lows of Diabetes

Chapter 7:
Highs and Lows of Diabetes

As a general rule, you can consider your child's diabetes to be reasonably well-controlled if her blood glucose level is within the target range most of the time, her A1C is within target range (see page 10), and she does not get severe symptoms of low blood glucose or frequent bouts of ketoacidosis (see page 7).

Sometimes insulin, food, and exercise are not balanced and your child may show signs of high or low blood glucose. Eating different amounts or different types of food or being more or less active than usual will affect your child's blood glucose levels. Differences in the way the body absorbs insulin or the presence of other hormones that respond to insulin may also cause blood glucose levels to be too high or too low.

Most of the time you'll be aware of situations that might cause high or low blood glucose—such as too much or not enough food, or too much or not enough exercise. However, it can happen for no apparent reason. Knowing how to identify high and low blood glucose levels, and what to do when they happen, can help you to act to protect your child's health.

HYPOGLYCEMIA (LOW BLOOD GLUCOSE)

Hypoglycemia is the most common problem in children with diabetes. Most of the time it is mild and can be easily treated. Food raises blood glucose levels while insulin and exercise lower them. Hypoglycemia can occur when the balance of insulin, food, and exercise is upset. Once an injection is given, the insulin can't be stopped. So, if too much insulin is available, blood glucose levels will drop too low. If a child uses a pump, it is possible to suspend the basal insulin or use a temporary reduced basal rate until blood glucose levels return to normal.

People with diabetes have to control their own blood glucose levels because their ability to regulate insulin is gone. Eating meals and getting insulin injections at regular times and snacking before exercise help to prevent glucose levels from dropping too low.

Hypoglycemia must be treated promptly to prevent blood glucose levels from getting so low that the brain is deprived of glucose. Too little glucose in the brain can cause severe symptoms, such as:

♦ sleepiness and unresponsiveness

♦ seizures

♦ unconsciousness

How Can I Tell If My Child's Blood Glucose Is Low?

The symptoms of low blood glucose may be different each time it happens. Sometimes your child may have no obvious symptoms. For these reasons, it is a good idea to teach a child with diabetes to tell you whenever she feels strange in any way.

In children under 3, crying, sleepiness, misbehavior, or crankiness may be signs that the child's blood glucose is low. Very young children can't tell you when they're not feeling well, so you need to be on the lookout for warning signs, such as pale, clammy skin, sweating, shakiness, sleeping, irritability, or crying. Frequent blood glucose tests can help to relieve anxiety when you aren't certain what is going on.

Researchers have shown that low blood glucose might continue to affect a child's learning ability for an hour or more after it has been

A teacher reported this experience with a usually pleasant and calm student. While waiting in the cafeteria line at lunch, the youngster became irritable and created a scene with a classmate for no apparent reason. The teacher knew the student to be generally polite and easygoing and this behavior was unusual. She pulled the student out of line, gave her a glass of orange juice, and walked her to the nurse's office where she checked her blood glucose. It was 50 mg/dl. She gave the student crackers and asked another student to get her lunch from the cafeteria and bring it to the nurse's office. By the time her lunch arrived, her blood glucose was 71 mg/dl and the student was her usual pleasant self again.

treated. When your child's glucose level is low it may not be the best time for her to take an important exam or give a presentation. This is another reason why it's a good idea to talk to your child's teachers about low blood glucose and do your best to avoid it on exam days.

Sometimes your child may feel nervous, anxious, or tired and think it's because of low blood glucose. The best thing to do if you or your child suspect that blood glucose is low is to check her blood sugar.

If the child has symptoms of low blood glucose but the blood test shows that glucose isn't low, repeat the test. She may be experiencing a fast drop in blood glucose without being in any danger of the more acute symptoms of hypoglycemia. Giving her a few crackers to eat should help the low feelings subside. In a few minutes she can return to her normal activities.

> " Low blood glucose might continue to affect a child's learning ability for an hour after it has been treated. "

If in doubt, treat. If you think your child may have low blood glucose but you can't do a blood test right away, give your child something with carbohydrates. The single treatment will not do any harm even if the child's glucose level is not low. If your child uses CGMS, there may be a lagtime between actual glucose and sensor readings. This is because of the time it takes for the interstitial fluid (read by the sensor) to reflect what is in the blood. Trust the feelings or symptoms your child has, and treat for low blood glucose.

Preventing Low Blood Glucose

It's important to prevent low blood glucose because frequent or unrecognized episodes can lead to more severe, potentially dangerous events. Low blood glucose can usually be prevented by:

♦ testing glucose levels regularly
♦ following the recommended meal plan
♦ making sure the insulin dose is correct
♦ eating extra snacks before exercise that is unplanned or more strenuous than usual

You may need to remind your child that testing blood glucose helps to make sure that the insulin dose and meal plan are right. Your child's insulin dose or meal plan may need to be changed if your child has frequent episodes of low blood sugar.

If you and your child are trying to keep her glucose levels near normal, you can expect that she will have mild episodes of low blood glucose occasionally. While not desirable, they are probably not dangerous and are easily treated.

It's essential for everyone who takes insulin to always carry carbohydrates for emergencies. Packages of glucose tablets, or juice boxes are useful because they are easy to carry. Glucose tablets are a first choice because they work quickly since they are already glucose and can be used immediately in that state. They are also easy to carry and come in a variety of flavors that most kids like. If you decide to use candy, be careful of the type. Avoid chocolate and caramel due to fat content that will retard absorption of sugar. Candy like Sweet Tarts, Smartees, or spice drops, etc., are a better choice. However, you might have to resort to whatever you can entice your young child to eat. It's also a good idea to pack a sandwich, cheese or peanut butter crackers, or some other food containing complex carbohydrate and maybe protein if your child is active and it is going to be a while until the next meal.

Treating Low Blood Glucose: Mild to Moderate

Low blood glucose needs to be treated quickly. The way to treat it is to give your child a sweet food like glucose tablets, fruit juice, regular (not "diet") soda, jelly, or raisins, followed by four crackers. A candy bar is not the best choice because its high fat content may not raise blood glucose quickly.

It may take 10 to 20 minutes for her blood glucose level to rise, depending on how much food is already in your child's stomach. If she isn't feeling better in 15 minutes, check her blood glucose level again. If it's still low, repeat the treatment.

A low blood glucose episode may occur just before a snack or a meal. If this happens, give your child glucose tablets or juice and see that she

The Rule of 15

If your child or teen feels low, check blood glucose. Is it in his target range?

If low, follow the rule of 15.

♦ Give him something with 15 grams of carbs (fast-acting carb like glucose gel or juice).

♦ Wait 15 minutes, then check his blood glucose.

If blood glucose is still too low, have him eat another 15 grams of carbs and check blood glucose again after 15 minutes. Once blood glucose level starts to get back in the target range, he should start to feel better.

Hint: Lots of people overtreat themselves when they feel low because they treat the symptoms and not the glucose level. This is especially true of many teens as they are often hungry and usually independent. Remind him that he may not feel better instantly after eating his 15 grams of carbs, but remember, the rule of 15. He may want to keep eating until he feels better but that might make his blood glucose levels shoot way up. Try to be patient and give it the full 15 minutes!

If he feels low, but can't check his blood glucose, he should go ahead and treat for a low blood glucose. When in doubt, it's always safer to get some food.

Hint: Try treating a low blood glucose with glucose tablets first. They might work faster than anything else as the body does not have to convert them from another form of carbohydrate to use it as glucose!

eats the snack or meal as soon as possible. If snack or mealtime isn't close, give your child a snack food containing complex carbohydrate and protein after the sweet food. Crackers with cheese or peanut butter, cereal and milk, or half a sandwich are good choices.

Treating Low Blood Glucose: Severe

A child who is very drowsy, unconscious, or unable to eat, drink, or swallow may be experiencing severe low blood glucose. When it occurs at night, children might have restless sleep, make strange noises, and if left untreated, can have a seizure. Please understand that it is not routine for children to become unconscious or have a seizure at night. This is very frightening for everyone and must be regarded seriously. Parents will address the concerns about night lows in different ways. Some will routinely check blood glucose levels through the night, or every night at 3 a.m. An insulin pump can be helpful at night because the basal rates can be turned down temporarily if you are concerned that blood glucose levels will drop. Some parents put baby monitors in the room, to listen for unusual noises. One family trained a guide-dog to react to hypoglycemia symptoms (and the dog could alert others).

It's best to be prepared for the worst case scenario, but most of the time, if your child is hypoglycemic, she will become uncomfortable and awaken, or will sleep through it as her low blood glucose will recover on its own due to a response from her own hormones. The problem is that you just can't count on that happening.

Glucagon is the treatment for severe hypoglycemia. It is normally made by the pancreas and one of its jobs is to raise blood glucose levels. If blood glucose levels drop dangerously low at any time, and your child is unable to eat, drink, or swallow a form of sugar, a glucagon emergency kit contains a syringe of glucagon that you can give your child to raise blood glucose. The full dose is 1 mg, but if your child is under 6 years old, you should give only half the dose, or 0.5 mg. If it happens that your child has symptoms of severe low blood glucose, do not put anything in your child's mouth if she is unconscious, as she could choke or clamp down on your fingers. If she can't or won't swallow, you will need to give her an injection of glucagon to raise blood glucose levels.

Treating Low Blood Glucose

Mild to moderate symptoms (child is alert and can swallow)

Treat right away with a sweet food:

- 1/2–3/4 cup orange or apple juice
- 1–2 glucose tablets or doses of glucose gel
- 2–4 LifeSavers (or similar product)
- 5 small gumdrops
- 1–2 Tbsp honey (DO NOT give to babies)
- 6 oz regular soda (not diet)
- 2 Tbsp cake icing (such as decorator icing gel in a tube)

Follow a few minutes later with:

- 2–4 soda crackers and 1 oz of cheese, OR
- 1 Tbsp peanut butter (or other complex carbohydrate and protein)

Severe Symptoms (very shaky, unconscious, or unable to eat)

- Treat immediately with an injection of glucagon. It should take 15–20 minutes for the glucagon to work. If the child doesn't respond, call your doctor immediately.

Keep a glucagon kit in strategic locations, such as Grandma's, if your child stays there frequently, or make sure you carry it with you. Review how to use it periodically and teach others. The injection usually takes effect within 10 to 20 minutes. If the child does not respond within that time, contact your doctor or take the child to an emergency room right away. A common side effect after taking glucagon is vomiting. Tell your doctor when you have needed to use glucagon—changes may need to be made in insulin doses. Do not hesitate to use it if you need to. Sometimes, when asked why parents did not use the kit, even when their child would not or could not eat or drink, they have commented "It says Emergency Kit, and it was not an emergency because he was awake." Keep a glucagon kit at home in a place everyone knows about, such as the refrigerator butter keeper. Check the expiration date on the kit periodically. Also keep a kit for travel in case of severe low blood glucose when you are on the road. Be sure that school personnel, babysitters, and others who take care of your child know where a kit is stored and how to use it.

Should My Child Wear a Medical ID Tag?

It's a good idea for everyone who has diabetes, including young children, to wear a medical identification tag at all times. These tags can save lives in an emergency. The kind of tag you choose will depend on your child's age and preference. It is most important that the tag be in a style your child will wear. For young children, ankle chains are probably the best choice. Neck chains are not suitable for infants and preschoolers, who are likely to play with the chains and may break them, get them caught, or choke on them.

A variety of colorful nylon or rubber bracelets are available for children. Teenagers may prefer a necklace-style chain. Sewing ID tags into the child's undershirts is another option. Soft, rubber bracelet ID's are colorful and popular with kids and teens alike. These can also be worn for most sports as metal or hard plastic ones must be removed as they have the potential to become imbedded in the flesh in contact sports.

Makers and styles of medical ID tags change frequently. Ask your diabetes educator or pharmacist for a current list of suppliers or see the *Diabetes Forecast Resource Guide*, published every January by the American Diabetes Association.

HYPERGLYCEMIA (HIGH BLOOD GLUCOSE)

Blood glucose levels can rise when your child gets too little insulin or too much food, or when she is less active than usual. Physical and emotional stress can also cause blood glucose levels to rise. Having a cold or sore throat, an injury, worrying about exams, family crises, poor insulin absorption, or going through the hormonal changes of puberty may all cause hyperglycemia. One of the most common reasons for high blood glucose is that kids and teens forget or intentionally do not take their bolus insulin.

Preventing and Treating Hyperglycemia

When blood glucose is high, there is an imbalance between the amount of food, exercise, and insulin present. Sticking to a meal plan is one of the best ways to keep within the target range. However, even then, sometimes blood glucose levels run high.

One of the most helpful strategies to prevent high blood glucose levels is to do frequent monitoring and keep records. Then you often can figure out how to prevent the high the next time. This will enable you to adjust your child's insulin dose, food intake, or exercise level to prevent symptoms from occurring. If your child uses a pump, it works best to regularly upload the information into the computer (all pump companies have this type of program) and review the data. You also will be able to see if your child or teen is regularly taking his bolus insulin, entering carbs, and taking the prescribed doses.

Unless a child is overweight and trying to shed pounds, it's not a good idea to cut down on food to lower blood glucose levels. Your child needs food to grow and develop normally. Her meal plan is designed to give her the nutrients she needs. Spacing meals and snacks farther apart may help if your child often gets high blood glucose, but talk this over with your doctor or diabetes educator before trying it. Mild exercise can also help to bring a moderately elevated (under 300 mg/dl) blood glucose down. (If there is a pattern of high blood glucose levels, insulin levels need to be adjusted.

KETOACIDOSIS AND DIABETIC COMA

Ketones are acid waste products that are created when the body burns fat to get the energy it needs. They build up in the blood and spill into the urine. Very high levels of ketones in the blood and urine lead to a condition called ketoacidosis.

Ketoacidosis is a very serious condition. Diabetic coma can be a result of severe or prolonged ketoacidosis. A person can have ketoacidosis without being in a coma, though. Untreated, ketoacidosis is life-threatening.

If your child is receiving enough insulin for her needs, she will not develop ketoacidosis even if her blood glucose level is high. Eating too much at dinner one night, or even a pile of candy will not cause ketoacidosis if the body has enough insulin to meet its needs. Blood glucose levels will undoubtedly rise, perhaps even extremely high, but if there is enough insulin in your child's system, ketones should not develop.

Ketoacidosis may occur if your child has very high blood glucose and is vomiting. Illness can cause other hormones such as adrenaline to be released, which then cause the need for extra insulin. These hormones help fight illness, but they also block the action of insulin. This is why you always give your child insulin when she is sick—even if she isn't eating well or vomiting.

Preventing and Treating Ketoacidosis

You can prevent ketoacidosis by checking urine or blood for ketones if blood glucoses are over 250 mg/dl and when your child is sick.

Ketoacidosis must be treated right away, possibly with intravenous (IV) fluids. Call your doctor immediately if your child has any of the symptoms listed in the box on the next page. A trip to the emergency room or a short hospital stay may be necessary.

REBOUNDING BLOOD SUGARS

You may notice that when your child has a low blood glucose, the next few blood glucose levels afterwards are high. You might think that your child ate too much or that you gave him too much to treat the low blood sugar, but in fact it is more likely a combination of factors that cause the high blood sugar. When blood glucose levels fall below normal, the body usually responds by producing extra adrenaline, glucagon, and other hormones that help the body deal with stress. These hormones cause the liver to stop storing glucose and release it into the blood and cause insulin not to work as well as usual.

Rebound is an abnormal increase in blood glucose that occurs after an episode of low blood glucose. This process is what helps to prevent your child's blood glucose level from dropping too low. Sometimes, the

When To Call the Doctor Immediately

Check with your child's doctor to learn when you should call. Always call right away if your child has any of the following problems. Your child may be developing ketoacidosis.

♦ moderate or high levels of ketones in the urine or blood

♦ dehydration (symptoms include sunken eyes; dry, cracked lips; dry mouth; skin that remains pinched up after it is pinched)

♦ persistent vomiting*

♦ any change in alertness or drowsiness

♦ labored breathing

♦ fruity-smelling breath (an odor like fruity chewing gum or nail polish remover)

♦ abdominal pain

If you can't reach the doctor, take the child to an emergency room right away.

*Vomiting can be caused by many illnesses. It is always a potentially serious problem for children with diabetes since it can cause ketoacidosis.

adrenaline and glucagon work for hours after blood glucose levels return to normal. This can cause high blood glucose several hours after an episode of low blood glucose.

One clue that this might be happening is a pattern of blood glucose tests that reads low, high, low, high, and so on. If you are checking for ketones, you might find that small amounts of ketones in the blood or urine are present. This can also be another clue. Reducing the insulin dose often helps fix the bouncing. Although the rebound effect does exist, it has less significance in daily control than previously thought. Some of the high blood glucose that follows a low might be from overtreatment of the low blood sugar with too much carbohydrate. Seek help from your health care provider if your child seems to be experiencing rebound.

DAWN PHENOMENON

People with diabetes frequently experience a rise in blood glucose levels very early in the morning. This increase is called the dawn phenomenon because it occurs at around 4 a.m. due to the release of hormones such as growth hormones. This occurs normally in everyone.

If your child is consistently waking in the morning with a high blood glucose, it would be smart to check his blood around midnight, then at 4 a.m. to see what is happening during the night. If the midnight number is okay, but the blood glucose rises from then until morning, more insulin may be needed. The dawn phenomenon can be addressed by increasing basal insulin at that time of night, if your child wears a pump.

HOW TO HANDLE SICK DAYS

Children with diabetes do not usually get sick more often than other children unless their blood glucose is persistently high. However, children with diabetes need special care when they get sick.

It may be helpful for you and your child's health care team to work out in advance a plan for handling sick days. The plan should include:

- ♦ phone numbers for reaching a doctor at all times
- ♦ guidelines for when it is important to call
- ♦ guidelines for adjusting insulin
- ♦ guidelines for checking blood glucose and adjusting your child's meal plan

Giving Insulin During Illness

Even when your child is ill, she will need insulin. It is intuitive to think that if your child is vomiting, and cannot eat, that you should withhold insulin. However, this is a very dangerous practice because when your child is vomiting, she actually might need more insulin than usual due to ketones. Your child should always take insulin, even if she is not eating well. Illness and stress can cause a need for more insulin. Children may need higher doses of rapid-acting insulin on sick days to lower blood glucose quickly. If your child is vomiting or not eating well, call your health care provider for advice on adjusting her insulin dose.

Helpful Hints for Sick Days

Your doctor can give you guidance tailor-made for your child, but the following general hints may be helpful.

♦ Write down phone numbers where you can reach a doctor at all times. Keep these numbers handy.

♦ Your child needs insulin every day and may need extra doses on sick days. Give insulin even if your child is not eating.

♦ Check blood glucose levels every 2 hours while your child is acutely sick and before meals, midnight and 4 a.m. as he recovers. Test urine for ketones.

♦ Try small meals and extra snacks. If your child has trouble eating, try special foods, even sweet ones that might appeal to your child. (When appetite is poor, it is more important to get some food into him, even if it is not the most healthy option.) Give your child plenty of fluids to drink.

♦ If your child is eating, give sugar-free fluids (such as sugar-free sodas or powdered drink mixes).

♦ If your child is not eating, give fluids that contain sugar and other nutrients (such as coke syrup, regular cola [not diet]), regular gelatin water (gelatin before it hardens), a Popsicle, sucker, clear broth, Gatorade, or Pedialyte).

Blood and Urine Testing

It's very important to check blood glucose levels and test urine for ketones more often than usual when your child is sick. The level of the blood glucose numbers is not as concerning as the presence of ketones. If blood glucose levels are above 250 mg/dl and your child is ill, check for ketones. If ketones are present, call your health care provider. The extra tests will help you and the health care provider decide how much extra insulin your child needs.

Test blood glucose before and 2 hours after the first bite of food, at midnight and 4 a.m. Your doctor might request that you check a blood glucose every 2 hours, and a urine ketone check every time your child urinates. If your child is vomiting or has large amounts of ketones in her urine, you may need to test both glucose and ketones every 2 hours. This stepped-up testing schedule should continue until ketones clear, blood glucose is back to normal, and your child feels better.

Eating During Illness

Try to keep your child on her regular meal plan as much as possible. She still needs food to balance her insulin. If your child has trouble eating regular foods, try some of the foods in the box on the next page. Small meals and extra snacks may be better than three big meals.

Encourage your child to drink lots of fluids, especially if she has a fever. It's very easy for a child to become dehydrated during illness. Dehydration robs the body of needed water and nutrients, can disrupt control of diabetes, and may contribute to ketoacidosis. The smaller the child, the greater the body surface area in relation to their size, and the more they can lose water due to sweating. It is much easier for a baby to become dehydrated than an adult.

If your child is eating, it's a good idea for her to drink water or sugar-free sodas, sugar-free powdered drink mixes, or sugar-free decaffeinated iced tea. If your child is not eating, is vomiting, has diarrhea, or has ketones in the urine, she needs fluids that contain carbohydrates and calories such as Pedialyte or low-sugar sports drinks.

Recommendations from the American Academy of Pediatrics note that foods with complex carbohydrates such as rice and cereal, lean meat, yogurt, fruit, and vegetables are foods of choice for children who are sick. For diarrhea, your child may need specially formulated products with electrolytes, found in your pharmacy. You will need to provide fluids that contain both carbohydrate (sugar) and sodium, such as Sprite, 7-Up, broth, or soup. Glucose tablets, Popsicles, and complex carbohydrates with salt (pretzels or crackers) are treatment for hypoglycemia.

Foods for Sick Days

These foods are well tolerated by most sick people. They may also be good substitutes when your child has an upset stomach or has trouble eating regular meals (for example, after getting braces).

- 1/2 cup (4 oz) regular soft drink with sugar (ginger ale or cola)
- 1/2 cup (4 oz) fruit juice (orange, grape)
- 1/2 twin-bar Popsicle
- 1 fruit (1 orange)
- 2 Tbsp corn syrup or honey (no honey for babies under the age of 1!)
- 1/4 cup (2 oz) sweetened gelatin
- 6 LifeSavers
- 1/2 cup (4 oz) ice cream
- 1/2 cup (4 oz) cooked cereal
- 1/4 cup (2 oz) sherbet
- 1/2 cup sweetened gelatin
- 2 cups broth-based soup, reconstituted with water
- 1 cup cream soup
- 3/4 cup (6 oz) regular soft drink with sugar (ginger ale or cola)
- 1/4 cup (2 oz) milkshake
- 1 slice toast
- 6 soda crackers
- 5 oz regular soft drink with sugar (ginger ale or cola)
- 1 cup yogurt
- 1 cup (8 oz) milk

INFECTIONS

If your child's glucose levels are in her target range, she should not get more infections than other children would. However, if she has frequent high blood glucose, she may be more likely to get infections. This is because bacteria grow well in a high-sugar environment, and bacteria-fighting cells do not work as well in a high-sugar environment. When blood glucose levels run high, it's easier to pick up an infection and harder to shake it off.

TAKING CARE OF TEETH AND GUMS

Children with diabetes usually do not have more dental problems than other children. They probably eat less candy and sugar-sweetened beverages than other children do, so they should have a lower risk of cavities.

However, gingivitis (inflammation of the gums) can be a long-term complication of diabetes. Gingivitis can lead to periodontitis, a more severe gum disease in which bone is lost and spaces develop between the gums and the teeth. Following healthy dental practices in childhood may prevent dental problems later on.

It's a good idea to brush teeth for a full 2 minutes twice a day and preferable to do it after every meal. If you treat low blood glucose with sweets at night, try to have your child brush her teeth afterward, or try to wash the sweet food down with water to rinse away sugar between the teeth. Do your best to avoid giving your child milk or juice at night. Take your child for regular dental checkups. If your child has red, swollen gums or any other dental problem, call your dentist immediately. It is never a good practice to give your child a bottle of milk in bed, or before sleeping without brushing teeth or rinsing.

If your child needs to have extensive work or dental surgery, ask your dentist to call your doctor so that the child's insulin dose can be adjusted on the day of the procedure and for a few days afterward. If your child's eating habits change after having dental surgery or getting braces, insulin will need to be adjusted. Stay in touch with your doctor or diabetes educator when your child is having dental work done. If you live in a rural area or place where the water does not have fluoride, your dentist can provide suggestions and also give fluoride treatments to prevent cavities.

THYROID DISEASE

The thyroid is a gland located in the neck. Hormones made by the thyroid gland help to control the way the body works (the metabolism).

Just as type 1 diabetes is an autoimmune disease, there is also a thyroid problem that is an autoimmune disease. The reasons why autoimmune attacks occur are not fully understood.

People who already have one autoimmune disease (diabetes) are at increased risk of developing another one. Therefore, people with type 1 diabetes are more likely than other people to develop thyroid disease.

There are two kinds of thyroid disease. Hyperthyroidism occurs when the thyroid gland makes too much of a hormone called thyroxin. This disease is not common in children with diabetes but can happen in adolescence. Hypothyroidism occurs when the thyroid does not make enough thyroxin. This disease is more common in children with diabetes than in other children.

When the thyroid gland is damaged by an autoimmune attack, it may get bigger and try to go on making normal amounts of thyroxin. This can cause a swelling in the front part of the neck called an enlarged thyroid gland or goiter. In time, the thyroid may no longer make normal amounts of thyroxin and symptoms of hypothyroidism appear. These symptoms include:

♦ weight gain
♦ feeling tired or sleeping more than usual
♦ feeling cold when others are not
♦ dry skin or hair loss
♦ constipation
♦ irregular menstrual periods.

If hypothyroidism is not treated it can affect a child's growth. Your child's doctor can check for hypothyroidism by feeling her thyroid gland and checking the level of thyroxin in the blood. This level should be checked at least once a year. Thyroid disease is easily treated with a pill containing thyroxin, the hormone that the thyroid gland no longer makes.

CELIAC DISEASE

Just as both type 1 diabetes and thyroid disease can have autoimmune causes, celiac disease is also more prevalent in children with diabetes. Celiac disease is an allergy to gluten, which is in wheat and wheat products, barley, and rye. Eating gluten can cause an inflammation in the lining of the intestines and the villa, which absorb nutrients. The inflammation can eventually damage small villa. Symptoms of celiac disease include constipation, diarrhea, abdominal pain, nausea, bloating, gas, or indigestion. Symptoms may not be specific, and some children have no symptoms at all. Often, the child's weight gain or growth is slower than expected. If left untreated, complications from chronic irritation to the bowel can follow, such as certain types of cancers, or irritable bowel syndrome.

The treatment for celiac disease is to follow a gluten-free diet, and when the diet is followed the intestinal villa return to normal and perform well. Growth should also be normal. Unfortunately, children who have both diabetes and celiac disease are even more limited in their diet, but generally get used to it and do quite well. A dietitian experienced with celiac disease and children will be your best resource.

COMPLICATIONS OF DIABETES

People who have diabetes for a long time may get other diseases that are caused by diabetes. These other diseases are complications of diabetes. It is rare for children to have complications; however, a child should have eye and urine micro testing five years after diagnosis.

Complications of diabetes can include blood vessel problems that lead to kidney disease, heart disease, eye disease, and nerve disease. Chronic high blood glucoses can damage the micro vessels in various body organs, and eventually, there is organ damage when the blood vessels leak. If it happens that the vessels in the back of the eyes leak, there are eye complications; in the kidneys, there are renal complications; in the cardiovascular system, heart attacks, strokes, and circulation problems; in the nervous system, inability to feel feet and hands, or to have an erection. The good news is that we now know that many of the complications can be prevented or delayed by tight control of blood glucose levels. Achieving tight control takes time, money, and energy. But the research has proven that the effort involved is worthwhile and gives people with diabetes hope for a healthy future.

Although complications of diabetes are rare in childhood, teaching your child healthy habits while she is young can help to prevent or reduce complications when she becomes an adult. For example, although diabetes foot problems are not a common issue in children or teens, learning to keep feet clean and taking care of blisters, injuries, cracks in the toes, or infections will be important later in life to reduce the risk of foot problems.

When your child is 10 years old and has had diabetes for 3–5 years, she should start seeing an eye specialist once a year for a dilated eye

Seventeen-year-old Susan had always had difficulty keeping her blood glucose in the target range. A well-meaning uncle tried to scare her: "Susan, you'll go blind like your grandmother." But instead of improving her diabetes care in response to this threat, Susan decided that if she was going to go blind there was no point in making an effort to maintain good glucose control. One approach might have been to talk with Susan openly about her problems dealing with her diabetes, help her understand that controlling blood glucose levels really can prevent complications once thought inevitable, and support her efforts to reach her goals. After some counseling, Susan realized that she felt that life was out of control, and that bad things happened (getting diabetes) and would continue to happen no matter what she did. Her counselor helped her see that although she had diabetes, she should have hope for a wonderful future, if she took charge of her diabetes. In time, she did learn to control her blood sugar and felt much more in control of herself and her future plans.

exam. School-performed eye tests are not sufficient as it is important that an eye doctor dilate the pupils to be able to see the back of the eyes.

Your doctor should periodically check for protein in your child's urine (a sign of kidney disease), and check her blood pressure and levels of fat in the blood (cholesterol, triglycerides, and other fats in the blood). If there are problems in any of these areas, they should be addressed by experts who work with children and teens. When caught early, complications of diabetes can sometimes be controlled with tight blood glucose control and expert care.

"Teaching your child healthy habits while she is young can help prevent complications in the future."

Children and teens should know that complications of diabetes do happen, and that they can be prevented. Prevention means tight blood glucose control, and early screening of problems. Children, teens, and adults should be seen by their diabetes professional every three months. Height, weight, urinalysis, and blood work for thyroid disease, cholesterol, protein in the urine, and eye exam are part of routine care.

The best way to deal with children and teens whose blood glucose levels are out of control is to work together in a non-judgmental way as a team. Diabetes care is tough and touches every aspect of life from sleeping, to eating, medications, record-keeping, managing exercise, and keeping supplies on hand. It is difficult for most adults and even the most dedicated children and teens cannot do it well without parental involvement. Kids whose parents stay involved in the care, supervising, guiding, and encouraging them, do well. Positive reinforcement and making changes one step at a time works for many parents and kids. Frightening youngsters into changing their behavior by threatening future complications has not been shown to be an effective way to impress young people to take care of themselves.

If your child is worried about getting complications in the future, it may help to have a talk with her health care provider. Your child may also benefit from counseling to help her adjust to living with diabetes.

As the parent of a child with diabetes, you too may have fears about the future. Feel free to discuss these fears with your health care provider. Your providers may be able to recommend a counselor who can help you to deal with these worries. Seeking help from a counselor is never a sign of weakness. On the contrary, it's a sign that you want to make life with diabetes the best it can be.

IF YOUR CHILD HAS TYPE 2 DIABETES

Most people are now quite aware of the obesity issues plaguing the U.S. and many other western countries. Over the past few decades, we have seen an enormous increase in the number of children and teens diagnosed with type 2 diabetes. In the past, it was rare for children or adolescents to get type 2 diabetes. Researchers and common sense point to societal changes as children eat out more frequently, eat more fast foods, watch more TV, play endless video and computer games, and spend less time in recreational activities. Today's children are heavier and more sedentary and family meal time and healthy well-balanced meals have declined.

In type 2 diabetes, the pancreas makes insulin but not enough and the body's cells can't use the insulin that is circulating. This is called insulin resistance. Insulin resistance means body cells can't get the glucose they need from the bloodstream. Insulin resistance gets worse with weight gain, and is improved by weight loss and exercise. Because the insulin does not work well, the body keeps making more of it, and people with type 2 diabetes will have high levels of insulin early in the course of the disease. Unfortunately, over a period of time, the cells that make insulin are not able to keep up, and high blood glucose levels are the result.

The signs and symptoms of type 2 in children are usually the same as the signs for type 1 diabetes (see page 6). Most adolescents with type 2 diabetes are overweight, eat a high-calorie diet, and don't get much exercise. They often belong to a family where other members also are obese and have type 2 diabetes.

People who have high levels of insulin in their system may have patches of darkened, velvety skin. This has been well recognized in people with type 2 diabetes. It often appears at the base of the neck, in the armpits, groin area, skin folds, and over flexor joints such as elbows, knees, and knuckles. Because the skin is actually thickened, it is not treatable externally, does not wash off, and is a sign that too much insulin is being produced.

There are several ways to take care of type 2 diabetes. The first step is to help the child lose weight by various weight loss strategies, healthy eating, and an exercise plan. If blood glucoses are still not well controlled, a medication, which is an oral pill, called Metformin might be added. The next step would be to add insulin as needed. The doctor will decide which kinds of insulin are best and how often they need to be taken. Sometimes, a long-acting insulin is all that is needed. Often adolescents with type 2 diabetes can go off insulin if blood glucose levels are lowered and they are successful in losing some weight or increasing their activity level.

Because the main problem is obesity, the main treatment is diet and exercise. A loss of excess body fat and improvement in exercise habits are the best way to treat insulin resistance. Unfortunately, making these lifestyle changes can be challenging. If your child has type 2 diabetes, you should work closely with the diabetes team, especially the dietitian.

It is now common for major pediatric centers to have programs for kids with type 2 diabetes, or those who are at risk. These programs have doctors, nurses, dietitians, psychologists, and exercise specialists who are trained to help in strategies for weight control and weight loss.

To find out what works best (insulin and/or pill) in controlling your child's blood sugar levels, your child will need to test her blood glucose. Your health care provider can tell when she will need to test. It will also be important for your child to have her blood tested for A1C levels.

Just like the child with type 1 diabetes, the child with type 2 diabetes is also at risk for getting infections and complications. In most cases, serious diabetes complications can be prevented. This is why keeping blood sugar levels as close to normal as possible is so important.

What Is Polycystic Ovarian Syndrome?

Polycystic Ovarian Syndrome (PCOS) is very common these days in young women and teens, and is related to type 2 diabetes. The causes of PCOS are unclear but are likely due to many factors and family history (genes) may be involved. It tends to run in families and, like type 2 diabetes, is often associated with being overweight. There is a problem in the feedback system of hormones that cause women's menstrual periods. When feedback signals don't work well, there can be too much or too little of certain hormones produced. When there is too much or too little of one hormone, others may try to fill the void, or shut themselves off. In this case, there develops an imbalance of male to female hormone.

It occurs when the hormones that cause a girl to have menstrual periods become unbalanced. Irregular periods, acne, male pattern hair growth, and infertility can result.

Signs of PCOS include weight gain or difficulty losing weight, irregular menstrual periods or no menstrual periods, male pattern hair growth on the face (sideburns, upper lip, chin), chest, midline hair on the stomach, back, or inner thigh, acne, and darkened skin at the base of the neck, skin folds, and knuckles.

Like women with type 2 diabetes, women with PCOS often have high levels of insulin and are at increased risk of type 2 diabetes, impaired glucose tolerance, and diabetes that occurs during pregnancy (gestational). They are also at increased risk for heart and blood vessel problems, including high blood pressure. PCOS affects their ability to become pregnant, their metabolism, and the health of heart and blood vessels.

Treatment for PCOS attacks the problem in different ways. Weight loss is important and will improve blood pressure, increased insulin production, and resistance to insulin. Enough weight loss might cause the symptoms to completely disappear. In teens, treating the problem of weight loss can become a family issue. When the whole family can engage in a healthy lifestyle program, the teen has the best chance of success.

Often, medications are added to weight loss efforts. Metformin is one of the medications often used (see above), which helps to improve insulin resistance. Birth control pills are also used to restore the female/male hormone imbalance.

CHAPTER 8:
As Your Child Grows Up

Chapter 8:
As Your Child Grows Up

G rowing up brings special challenges and rewards for both children and parents. Growing up with diabetes is an additional challenge, and growing up healthy brings special rewards, not only for your child but also for you. All parents worry about their children, but it's natural for you to worry a little more about your child with diabetes. By presenting an overview of situations you may encounter as your child grows up, this chapter may help you to worry a bit less.

WHEN YOUR BABY HAS DIABETES

With good medical care, babies with diabetes grow and develop into healthy, active children. Your doctor and other health care providers can help you to adjust insulin and food intake so your infant will grow and gain weight normally. You can expect your baby to roll over, sit up, crawl, and talk the same time as other babies.

If your baby is hospitalized, you may find that he briefly loses some of the skills he had developed or goes back to acting the way he did at a younger age. For example, an infant who drank from a cup may insist on a bottle for a while after coming home from the hospital. This behavior is not caused by diabetes. Any child who undergoes a stressful experience like being hospitalized may cope by seeking comfort in familiar things like a pacifier. Once your baby settles down at home again, he will soon regain any lost skills and continue to develop normally.

If you are breast feeding, you can continue to do so. You should talk to your nurse or diabetes educator regarding the details of your baby's feeding schedule and supplemental formula.

How Can I Tell If My Baby Has Low Blood Glucose?

Parents are usually most worried about low blood glucose in infancy because babies can't communicate that they feel strange. You will need to learn to look for signs like these that may tell you your baby's glucose is low:

♦ sweating, clammy
♦ pale skin
♦ irritability
♦ tiredness
♦ shaking
♦ crying
♦ restlessness at night
♦ bluish color around the lips

Regular blood glucose tests are very important in babies. Your doctor or diabetes educator can help you learn to do these tests. Blood may be taken from heels, or toes if little fingers become tender from too many fingersticks. It is always a good idea to treat your baby if you are unsure whether he is having a low. When in doubt, treat.

Treating a Baby for Low Blood Glucose

1. Give the baby a sugary drink (such as apple juice, sugar water, or glucose gel). This should have an effect within 20 minutes.
2. Follow with formula or milk. If the baby is eating solids, you may give cereal, vegetables, or meat instead of milk.
3. If the baby won't eat or if symptoms don't improve, give a glucagon injection and call your doctor. Make sure you already have instructions from your doctor on how much glucagon to give your baby. Half the usual dose of glucagon (0.5 mg) is suggested for infants.
4. Do not give honey to babies under 1 year of age because of the risk of botulism. Botulism spores can be found in some honey products.

Illnesses in Infancy

Infants with diabetes don't get infections, colds, or diarrhea more than other babies. If your baby with diabetes does get sick, be sure to follow your doctor's sick-day guidelines. Sick-day guidelines for babies are the same as those for older children (see How to Handle Sick Days, page 118); however, a baby can become very sick more quickly than an older child can because an infant becomes dehydrated faster. Symptoms of dehydration include:

♦ sunken eyes
♦ dry, cracked lips
♦ dry mouth
♦ skin that remains pinched up after being pinched

Because of the risk of dehydration, make sure your baby continues to take in fluids when he is sick and call your doctor immediately. It's very important to check for ketones frequently when your baby is sick.

Babies with diabetes who have diarrhea should be treated in the same way that any other child with diarrhea would be treated. Give liquids with electrolytes or foods that contain both carbohydrate and small amounts of sodium or salt (e.g., crackers). Your baby may need less insulin when he has diarrhea or another illness that causes him to eat less than usual. Talk to your doctor about how to adjust insulin during illness.

If Your Baby Won't Eat

All babies go through stages when they won't eat; however, babies with diabetes need food to balance their insulin. If your baby won't eat, and isn't yet on solid food, you can try offering other fluids (like juice, sugar water, or Pedialyte). If the baby is on solids, try offering a different food, or try fluids.

If your baby refuses both solids and fluids, wait 10 minutes and try again. Offering small amounts frequently may be helpful. It's never a good idea to force your infant to eat. You may have to settle for feeding the baby any foods (or fluids) that he likes, such as ice cream, pudding, tapioca, or cookies. For a young child with diabetes, this is always preferable to no food.

If Your Baby Is Vomiting or Has Diarrhea

1. Call the doctor right away.
2. Begin to give the baby small amounts of sugary fluids, such as apple juice, sugar water, gelatin water (gelatin before it hardens), or Pedialyte.
3. You will need to check for ketones when your baby is sick. Because infants can easily become dehydrated, and of course do not "pee" on demand, it will be important that you obtain a meter that reads levels of blood ketones and also check blood glucose levels often.

Coping When Your Baby Has Diabetes

Caring for an infant with diabetes can be difficult and stressful. It's natural for parents to worry about their baby having low blood glucose or not eating, or about giving the baby insulin injections. Insulin pumps are now most often used for very young children because of the accuracy of insulin delivery in extremely small doses.

For your own mental well-being, it's important that you be able to take a break from caring for your baby for an afternoon, an evening, or a weekend. If you and your spouse are sharing the care, you need uninterrupted time together. Find a person you trust—a friend, an aunt, or a grandparent —who can care for your baby while you take a break. This caregiver will need general training in diabetes care and an understanding of your baby's care routine. Your doctor, dietitian, or diabetes educator may be able to suggest additional sources of support when you become very stressed. Asking for help is never a sign of weakness. You have a lot to cope with. (See Asking for Help, page 186).

YOUR PRESCHOOLER WITH DIABETES

Parents of a preschooler with diabetes may have the same feelings of anxiety and helplessness that parents of infants have. Low blood glucose can still be a big worry. You still need to be on the lookout for signs of low blood glucose (see page 8) because your child can't always tell you how he is feeling. Frequent blood glucose checks are a good way to reassure yourself that your child is alright.

How To Help a Child Accept Injections and Testing

Insulin injections and regular blood glucose tests are very important to your child's diabetes care, but the needles and fingersticks can be frightening to a preschooler. An insulin pump may be a great way to manage an active pre-schooler as it can deliver insulin precisely in tiny doses.

It may help to say to your child: "Yes, I know this pinches and I'm sorry," and "You're being very brave." Let the child choose which finger to use for the fingerstick or where to give the insulin injection. Feeling that he has some control over the situation may help to ease the child's anxiety. An adhesive bandage to cover the wound and a hug or a kiss when it's over may be all it takes to smooth things out.

You may want to try using stickers or star charts as incentives to help your child accept finger sticks and injections. Explain that every time he has a finger stick or an injection, he will earn a star or sticker. When he has 20 stars, he can plan a special treat like a trip to the zoo or another fun activity.

Young children may try to delay finger sticks and injections. They'll say, "Wait just one more minute and I'll be ready." But one minute soon becomes 15 and the child is late for preschool. One solution to this problem is to use a cooking timer.

> "Praise your child for being brave and holding still while you give the injection."

Set the timer for 10 minutes and explain that if the child has the finger stick or injection before the bell rings, he will earn a star. But if the procedure isn't done when the bell rings, he won't get a reward.

Praise your child for being brave and holding still while you give the injection. Try not to scold him for moving during the finger stick or for being late for an injection.

At times, even praise and the offer of rewards may not help. Your child just won't cooperate. Preschoolers may find it hard to understand why they need injections, especially if they don't feel sick. If this happens, you may have to hold the child or get someone to help you give

Four-year-old Larry was terrified of getting his insulin injections. His mother reported that he avoided going to bed at night because he associated waking up in the morning with getting an injection. He woke up during the night with nightmares about the injection. Every morning his parents chased him through the house to give him his insulin and often had to search for him under the bed or in the closet.

One day, Larry's mother began including his favorite stuffed animal in the procedure. Before giving Larry his insulin, she went through the entire routine with the toy, including placing a Band-Aid over the injection site. Finally, Larry began giving his "bunny with diabetes" the injection. Through play, he was able to express feelings that he couldn't express in words. Eventually, he got over his fear of injections.

the injection. This is never pleasant, but your child needs to get insulin regularly. Afterward, it may be helpful to hug your child and explain that you have to give the injections "to keep you well."

Children often express their frustrations and worries through play. Having your preschooler give an injection to a favorite doll or stuffed animal may help him express his fears.

How Can I Get My Child to Eat Regularly?

Getting a youngster with diabetes to eat properly can be just as challenging as giving finger sticks and insulin injections. Young children often try to take control at mealtimes. One of the most effective ways of handling a child who fusses at meals may be to not make an issue of eating or not eating. If the child rejects a meal, offer something else. If that's rejected, try offering orange juice or a piece of fruit. Give rapid-acting insulin based on what your child actually eats (give it after the meal). The meal can be offered again later. Watch carefully for signs of low blood glucose if your child is going through a fussy eating phase.

Don't let your child prolong meals so that breakfast, snack, and lunch all seem to run together. Allow a certain amount of time for meals. When the time is up, the meal is over. Without this kind of discipline, your child

Two-year-old Laura was the youngest of 3 children. School mornings for the family were hectic. Laura got her insulin injection and her breakfast while her mother was busy getting the older children ready for the school bus. Although Laura liked her breakfast cereal, she never finished eating it. Because she had not eaten enough food, Laura always had low blood glucose before lunch. After talking with the diabetes educator about this, Laura's mother changed the family's morning routine. Now she waits until the older children have left for school before giving Laura her insulin injection. Then she makes sure that Laura eats her breakfast and has a midmorning snack to prevent low blood glucose.

will be nibbling constantly and his blood glucose will always be out of control.

When your child is not eating well, try not to nag or physically force him to eat. Usually, this kind of pressure will often increase the child's resistance. Instead, try providing positive rewards for behavior you want to encourage. Sometimes when children are not in the mood for eating an entire meal, they may be willing to drink something. A carbohydrate-containing beverage, such as milk or flavored milk, may help prevent low blood glucose later on.

It's common for children to want to eat nothing but peanut butter sandwiches for days on end and then to suddenly switch to wanting nothing but hot dogs. As long as the current favorite food is reasonably healthy, it's okay to let your child eat it as many days in a row as he wants. It has been shown that children self-regulate their nutrition.

What If My Child Needs To Be Hospitalized?

Being hospitalized for newly diagnosed diabetes can be very stressful for a child. It can be scary and confusing. The child may think that having diabetes or being in the hospital is a punishment for being bad. It's important to reassure your child that none of these things is his fault.

Your child may be anxious or afraid about being away from home. It helps if you can stay with your child while he is in the hospital. Children's units will let parents stay with their children. If you can't stay, it's important to try to tell your child why, and perhaps find a substitute. Be honest about when you will be back. Leaving the child's favorite toy or blanket can help to ease his anxiety.

For many parents, the period of their child's hospitalization is a time to learn (in a safe environment) as much as they can about their new responsibilities as the parents of a child with diabetes. If your child is not hospitalized when he is diagnosed, you may be able to attend an outpatient program about diabetes care for parents. In either case, diabetes educators will provide help and advice as you learn to give insulin injections and do blood tests.

Daycare and Preschool

When you decide to send your young child to preschool or daycare, the decision of where to go is sometimes difficult. Although any setting that receives any kind of federal funding cannot discriminate about taking a child with a chronic illness or disability, liability concerns, staffing issues, and insurance policies often dictate whether or not a child is accepted into a daycare facility. You will be most concerned about your child's safety, and it is necessary that you ensure that all staff members are informed and knowledgeable about diabetes and your child's individual care plan. You'll want to pay special attention to educating the staff about hypoglycemia: how to recognize the symptoms and provide treatment.

This will involve carefully screening and selecting a daycare facility, educating the staff, putting together a diabetes care plan that includes courses of action based on blood glucose readings, and keeping in close communication with the staff. Usually after the staff members understand the issues of diabetes and become comfortable with how to care for your child, they will welcome him.

THE SCHOOL-AGE YEARS

Children ages 6 to 12 usually have a lot of energy and are eager to learn and do things. They have a vivid imagination, a conscience, and the ability to share and cooperate. They display energy in horseplay, teasing, schoolwork, games, and fantasy. They have an increasing desire for

Sample Daycare or Preschool Care Plan

1. When to do a blood glucose test

   ◆ She says, "I'm low," especially if during or after exercise.

   ◆ If she has symptoms of hypoglycemia.

2. What to do based on your child's blood glucose reading (this is an example only and should be adapted to your child's needs)

   ◆ 60 mg/dl or under. Give two glucose tablets, followed immediately by food containing 30 grams of carbohydrate. If she doesn't respond or glucose levels don't rise within 20 minutes, telephone parent for further instructions.

   ◆ 61 to 100 mg/dl. Give one glucose tablet. If a meal or snack comes within 30 minutes, she can wait. Otherwise, give her a snack including carbohydrates and protein, such as cookies and milk.

   ◆ 101 to 140 mg/dl. She is fine. If exercise is planned before a meal or snack, she must have a snack before participating.

   ◆ 141 to 300 mg/dl. She's fine, but higher than we'd like. No action is necessary.

   ◆ Over 301 mg/dl. Her blood glucose is too high. She should receive a bolus of insulin on her insulin pump or with a syringe. She can also be encouraged to drink water or other non-caloric fluids. Allow bathroom use, if needed. She needs to check her urine or blood for ketones. If ketones are present, the parents or diabetes team should be called for advice.

   If the blood sugar remains low despite treatment and the student is not thinking clearly, the parents or diabetes care team should be called. Following an episode of hypoglycemia, it can take several hours to fully recover.

independence, but they still want their parents' protection and authority.

Starting school or moving on to middle school is a new challenge that may cause a child with diabetes to feel insecure at times. He is meeting a lot of new people and facing new demands such as increased homework and competitive school sports. He may become anxious because his parents aren't always with him. Parents, in turn, may try to overprotect a child with diabetes. When the child starts going to school, it may be the first time the parent has been separated from the child.

> "You can help your child by encouraging him to lead as normal a life as possible while still taking care of himself."

For these reasons, it may be hard for a child with diabetes to be as independent as other children his age. Balancing a child's needs for independence and protection is hard. Yet you help your child most by encouraging him to lead as normal a life as possible while still taking good care of his diabetes.

If you have concerns about how to balance your child's needs for independence and protection, you may want to discuss your feelings with your doctor or diabetes educator. School-age children are often ready to do more of their diabetes care than their parents think they can handle. However, they generally feel more secure when a parent or another adult, such as the school nurse or a teacher, supervises and supports their diabetes care efforts.

Ideas on Handling the Rough Times

As children begin to develop their own identities and separate from their parents, they may go through periods of struggle against adults. This is a normal part of growing up, but the struggle may be harder for a child with diabetes who has to take insulin, check blood and urine all the time, and follow a meal plan.

There are no easy solutions. It may help to talk with your child about his concerns. Talking over his feelings about having diabetes can help to ease his tension, and also help you understand what he is going through.

Encourage other family members to talk to your child and offer their support. Sometimes your child with diabetes will benefit from talking with another adult, such as a favorite teacher, school counselor, doctor, nurse, social worker, or minister.

Learning about diabetes and taking on self-care tasks may help your child come to terms with having diabetes. Often when children are diagnosed with diabetes very young, they never learn basic information about the disease. Understanding how the disease works and why they need to take insulin, checking their blood glucose, and learning what foods affect their glucose levels can help children accept having diabetes. As your child grows and develops, both you and he will need continuing education about diabetes. It can take years for a child or adult to come to terms with having diabetes. Be patient and loving with your child as he learns to handle this difficult challenge.

Diabetes and Your Child's Friends

When children start school, their relationships with their friends become very important to them. Your child's attitude about diabetes can influence his friends' attitudes. Every child's personality is different and it is smart to respect and work with your child's style of coping. Some kids are private while others are much more extroverted. If your child accepts diabetes positively, it's likely that his friends will do the same. You can help your child to develop a positive attitude by demonstrating your love, support, and understanding.

Your child's friends may be fearful because they lack information about diabetes. Encourage your child to be open about the disease with his friends. A child's willingness to be open about diabetes will depend on his personality. Sometimes a child with diabetes feels sensitive about being different from his friends because he has to take insulin, test his blood glucose, and follow a meal plan.

Some children have checked their blood glucose or given themselves an insulin injection or pretend injection for show-and-tell. Older children have presented science projects on diabetes and its care. It's important to mention that a child who is sensitive or shy about having diabetes may not wish to draw attention to himself in this way. Understanding your child's personality will help you to handle these situations in the way that works best for him.

Communicating With Your Child's School

Your child's teachers, the school nurse, and the principal of your child's school all need to know about his diabetes. When your child starts school, changes schools, or has a new teacher, it's a good idea for parents to ask for a meeting with all of these people. This way, everyone hears the same information at the same time and their questions can be answered. Having a written plan that includes important phone numbers is also helpful. Ask the school staff to inform you whenever there is a change to the school schedule that affects your child's meal times or exercise routine, so you can plan ahead.

Your School's Legal Responsibilities

The level of health care assistance available at your child's school will vary. Few schools today employ a full-time school nurse. Often, one school nurse covers an entire school district. Schools often rely on the school secretary or a health aide to provide emergency health care.

Under federal law, diabetes is considered a disability, and it is illegal for schools to discriminate against a person with a disability. Federal law also requires that anyone with a disability have full access to public programs, which include public schools. In addition, federal law entitles children with diabetes to special education services if they need them.

When a school is notified that a child has diabetes, it must do an evaluation of the child's special needs. This might require obtaining medical information from the child's doctor or health care team. The school must prepare a plan that outlines how the child's special health care needs will be met so that he has an equal opportunity to take part in all school programs. The school must consult you, the child's parent, about the plan, and it cannot alter the plan without your consent. A school staff member must be designated to be responsible for implementing the plan, and other school staff must know what the plan requires them to do. The plan should be updated every year.

You will find that most schools are very cooperative and want to help. If, however, your child is having problems and the school is not supportive, you will need to step in. Most laws that protect school children with diabetes have been made because of parents who insisted on having a safe and healthy setting for their children. If you have problems or feel that your child is not being treated fairly, contact the American Diabetes Association's (ADA) Government Relations Division for help. Your local ADA chapter can help guide you. Resources for you are listed in the back of this book and are important for you to use for your children in school. Learn your rights that fall under the Americans with Disabilities Act, and the importance of having a 501c3 plan of care.

Checking Blood Glucose at School

Parents and school personnel should meet at the beginning of each school year to put together an individualized diabetes care plan for your child (See Diabetes Care Plan For School, page 147). Children in school should test blood glucose before lunch, and before taking part in a strenuous sport like basketball or football, at the very least. Many kids will also check mid-morning and mid-afternoon.

Decide with school staff and your child where the best place is to test. Find out which school staff member is responsible for helping your child to do a blood test, and ask him or her to record the test result. This will help you to monitor patterns in your child's glucose levels. Every school district seems to handle things a bit differently, but the bottom line is that your child is safe and cared for, and that every other child is safe from being pricked accidentally with a needle or lancet.

Your child may feel uncomfortable about doing blood tests at school, or it may really disrupt his school routine to have to do the tests. If this is the case, ask your diabetes educator for advice about how often testing is necessary and how to fit it in during a busy school day.

What If My Child Has Low Blood Glucose at School?

Your child's teachers and other school staff, such as the secretary, health aide, or school nurse (if there is one) need to know the signs of low blood glucose. Subtle signs can be missed unless the school staff is well informed. For example, these behaviors may be signs of undetected low blood glucose:

♦ midmorning sleepiness
♦ lack of attention in class just before lunch or in mid-afternoon
♦ complaints of a headache after gym class.

Most elementary school teachers can treat your child in the classroom by giving him a glucose tablet (if he is not treating the episode on his own). Be sure to stress that your child should not be sent to the nurse's office alone. A friend should go along in case low blood glucose causes your child to become dizzy or confused.

It's a good idea to give a supply of glucose gel, glucose tablets, crackers, or small juice boxes to your child's teacher, as well as to your child, for emergencies. You may want the gym teacher to have a supply as well. Someone in your child's school should be prepared to give a glucagon injection, if necessary. This could be a nurse, teacher, or designated assistant. Many school districts do not allow school personnel to give glucagon injections. Find out what your school district's policy is when you meet with your school's staff.

Handling Snacks at School

Your child may need to eat one or more snacks during the school day. You may decide to send a supply of snacks to be kept at the school or to pack snacks daily with the child's lunch.

Your child should probably also eat a snack before gym class. If gym is right after a meal, the snack should be eaten after the class rather than before. Crackers with peanut butter or cheese, pretzels, or apples are excellent snacks.

Some teachers have used classroom snack time to teach children about healthy eating. Many early development programs are now

Diabetes Care Plan for School

Every child with diabetes should have a diabetes care plan at the beginning of every school year. This information should be shared with school personnel so they are prepared if they need to assist your child.

- ♦ Target blood glucose levels
- ♦ Food, insulin, and testing schedules
- ♦ How to handle exercise
- ♦ Symptoms of high and low blood glucose
- ♦ When and where to test blood glucose
- ♦ Plan for treating low blood glucose

prohibiting candy and desserts for snacks, and encouraging fresh fruits and vegetables. For carbohydrates, they might serve popcorn or a cereal mix. This helps the child with diabetes feel like they're fitting in with the group and it also teaches healthy eating to all, and may introduce them to new foods.

What If My Child Has High Blood Glucose at School?

It's important to explain to the staff of your child's school the signs of high blood glucose. It may be helpful to also explain that when your child's blood glucose is running a bit high, he may need to make extra trips to the bathroom or the water fountain.

The school should also have doctor's orders for checking for ketones if blood glucose levels are high. There should be an action plan for who to call, and what to do with the information.

You may want to ask your child's teacher or the school nurse to tell you when your child has signs of high blood glucose. These signs may indicate that your child's insulin dosage needs to be adjusted.

School Lunches and Parties

Many schools make lunch menus available ahead of time, giving you and your child a chance to plan. (Help Your Child Accept a Meal Planning? page 88.)

When you talk with the staff at your child's school, you may want to mention that your child must try to avoid eating fatty foods and sweets most of the time. You can also explain that there will be times when he will be allowed to join in and eat what the other kids are eating, and then figure out a way with the school how to communicate this information. This will help them to be sensitive to your child's needs at special events or parties. But teachers and other school staff should not be expected to keep an eye on what your child eats every day.

> "Kids with diabetes should be able to eat the same food as the other kids as long as they prepare for the party with extra insulin."

School parties can be hard on children with diabetes. Your child will want to eat the same party food that the other children are eating, and they can. Ask the teacher to let you know when a party is planned and suggest that he or she also speak to the parents of the child who is having the party. Some teachers will encourage all parents to bring party foods that all the children can eat. If you have time and know ahead what's happening in school, you might send in a bag of air-popped popcorn or pretzels so the children have some low-fat options during the party. It is fine for the child to eat cake or a cupcake, just make sure that the child takes extra insulin, if needed. Kids with diabetes should be able to eat the same food as the other kids, as long as they prepare for the party with extra insulin and make sure she doesn't overindulge (See Holidays and Parties, page 92.)

Will My Child Have To Miss a Lot of School?

Your child with diabetes should not have to miss school more than other children. Frequent absences from school due to diabetes are a signal that your child's diabetes is not being controlled as well as it should be.

The cafeteria staff at 10-year-old Drew's school knew about his diabetes and wanted to be helpful. Every day when Drew bought his lunch, a cafeteria aide would check his tray to make sure he selected a healthy lunch. Drew, embarrassed by this, stopped eating his lunch. As a result, he started having low blood glucose in the early afternoon. When Drew's mother found out what was happening, she arranged to meet with the school staff, thanked the cafeteria aides, but asked them not to check on Drew's food choices. Drew was then able to eat his lunch without embarrassment and began the huge responsibility of taking care of himself.

Frequent absences may also be a warning sign that your child is struggling emotionally. Sometimes a child may try to use diabetes as an excuse to avoid going to school. If this happens, you may want to seek advice from a doctor, social worker, school counselor, psychologist, or psychiatrist. (See Asking for Help, page 186.)

DIABETES CAMP

Going to camp can be a great experience for any child. Camps geared to children with diabetes make sure that the experience is safe and healthy. Most diabetes camps have these goals:

♦ giving children the opportunity to meet other children who have diabetes
♦ helping children to be more self-sufficient by teaching them about diabetes and self-care

Each diabetes camp has its own way of teaching children about diabetes. Some camps use schoolroom-type lectures. Others have a much more informal structure.

Going to camp seems to help most children with diabetes. They learn more about their condition and often learn to give their own insulin injections for the first time. At camp, children with diabetes meet other children who share the same problems. They come away with new information about products, managing their insulin, healthy eating, and their own special needs in a camping situation. After leaving camp, children often become pen pals and continue to share their feelings and fears.

Camp can provide an opportunity for children to learn independence and assume self-care tasks. Parents can feel comfortable knowing that the camp staff is trained to handle problems related to diabetes. For a complete list of camps for children with diabetes and other activities, contact the local chapter of the American Diabetes Association or 1-800-diabetes.

DIABETES AND YOUR CHILD'S WEIGHT

Children, especially teenagers, are often very concerned about their appearance and may want to know how diabetes can affect it. Children with diabetes do not look any different from other children; however, if diabetes is not well cared for, it may affect a child's height and weight. Thyroid disease may also cause growth problems (see page 123). Your child's doctor should monitor his height and weight carefully.

Sudden weight loss or lack of weight gain or growth can be a sign of uncontrolled diabetes. When the body doesn't have enough insulin, it breaks down fat to obtain energy and eliminates more water than usual, causing weight to drop. When body cells don't have enough insulin, growth is slowed. Once your child's blood glucose levels are brought under control, he should regain the lost weight and grow normally.

If Your Child Wants to Lose Weight

Losing weight can be hard for a plump child or teen with diabetes because he must eat regularly to cover insulin. A child with diabetes cannot go on a crash diet.

Sometimes teenagers with diabetes decide that losing weight is more important than controlling blood glucose levels. If a teen skips meals or cuts calories without reducing insulin, he can end up with severe low blood glucose. Teens may also try to lose weight by cutting down on insulin, which can cause severe high blood glucose.

If a child with diabetes wants to lose weight, it is best to get help from a doctor and/or a dietitian. Weight loss through a low-calorie diet that limits fat intake, provides the right nutrients, and controls blood glucose levels may take longer, but it will be safer. When a lower-calorie diet is recommended, it's important to reduce insulin. Getting more exercise is often a helpful weight-loss strategy.

Fad diets and diet pills are very popular, especially among teenage girls. Fad diets can be harmful because they may not provide enough nutrients. In people with diabetes, a fad diet can upset blood glucose control.

Over-the-counter diet pills may work for a short time for weight loss, but many people soon regain weight. Because diet pills can cause dizziness, nervousness, anxiety, sleeplessness, and other side effects, they are not recommended for children and teens. Joining a weight-loss program can be helpful. Teens, especially, seem to do better at weight loss in a group with other teens.

BROTHERS AND SISTERS

Siblings can be a great asset to a child with diabetes. Because brothers and sisters usually know each other well and notice unusual behavior, a sibling may be the first to pick up signs of low blood glucose.

Because a youngster with diabetes gets a lot of attention, brothers and sisters may sometimes feel anxious or neglected. Seeing their brother or sister with low blood glucose can be frightening, especially for younger siblings, who may fear that the child with diabetes will die. Brothers and sisters may think that their angry feelings or bad thoughts caused their sibling to get sick. They may also be afraid that it will happen to them. These fears can be addressed through conversation, reassurance, play, or professional counseling. Consult your doctor, social worker, diabetes educator, or clergy for help if your other kids are having trouble dealing with diabetes in the family.

It is important to talk these fears over with children and reassure them that they did not cause their sibling's diabetes. Once they are about 5 or 6 years old, children can take part in educational sessions about diabetes and can even be encouraged to help with the care of their sibling with diabetes.

Amy, a teenager with newly diagnosed diabetes, was having a hard time accepting her insulin injections. Every morning she created a scene by refusing her insulin. The whole family's attention was on her, including that of her adoring 3-year-old brother. No one realized how her scenes were affecting him until one morning he began crying and told his mother to give him the injection instead. When Amy realized that her behavior was affecting her brother, she began to understand how her behavior was influencing everyone in the family, and maturely accepted the shots.

Brothers and sisters may be afraid of getting diabetes themselves. The chance that this will happen is very slim. Studies show that about 5 out of every 100 siblings of a child with type 1 diabetes may get diabetes by age 30. To put it more positiviely, there is a 95% chance that a sibling will not get type 1 diabetes.

How Brothers and Sisters Can Help

Brothers and sisters can be taught the signs and symptoms of low blood glucose and can help parents watch for these signs in the child with diabetes. For example, a sibling who shares a bedroom with the child with diabetes can be asked to tell parents if he hears his brother making funny noises or sleeping restlessly. Siblings who are mature enough can help with blood testing or with giving insulin injections.

But brothers and sisters are not substitute parents. Although they may be very willing to help when their sibling with diabetes needs them, they should not be forced to assume the burden of caring for their sibling.

Planning Meals for the Family

It's a good idea for the whole family to eat the same meals instead of serving a separate meal for the child with diabetes. This helps the child with diabetes to feel part of the family. Other family members benefit by learning healthy eating habits. When siblings understand the dietary needs of the child with diabetes, they can help him to select healthy foods.

Fourteen-year-old Anne and her 12-year-old sister Wendy played on a softball team together. One day during a game Anne noticed that Wendy was stumbling a lot and throwing the ball poorly. She pulled her sister off the field and told the coach that Wendy needed to check her blood sugar. She was low, so she gave her sister glucose tablets and crackers to eat. Additionally, although the coach had been told what to look for regarding symptoms of low blood sugar, he now had a better picture so he could recognize the problem if it happened again.

Some parents may feel that they are punishing their other children by not having sweets in the house. They buy foods for the other children that the child with diabetes can't eat. This is very hard on the child with diabetes, who may not have enough self-control to refuse to eat candy or other treats. As one teenage girl remarked, "When cookies are sitting there, it's hard not to want them."

All children need to know that following a healthy meal plan is not a punishment, but a lifelong habit that will help them to stay well and keep them from being fat or getting cavities. The meal plan for your child with diabetes can be flexible enough to include occasional sweet treats. Parents may also suggest to other children that they eat sweets occasionally when they are out with their friends instead of at home.

YOUR TEEN WITH DIABETES

The teen years are often a challenging time for both youngsters and parents. As teenagers move toward adulthood they go through many physical and emotional changes. Their increasing maturity and desire for greater independence can affect their diabetes care and strain relationships with their parents. When life is going great and a child or teen is doing well socially and emotionally, his diabetes control might be quite reasonable. When things aren't going so well, his blood glucose levels might run high or low or become extremely variable.

For the teenager with diabetes, having to take insulin, test blood glucose regularly, and stick to a meal plan can all compound the normal difficulties of puberty. It's tempting for many teens to ease up on diabetes care and try to act like everyone else.

The teenage years are a period of developing a new identity. Many teens try to distance themselves from their families. Teens with diabetes may try to show their independence by:

♦ refusing to do blood tests
♦ making up false test results
♦ bingeing on sweets or fatty foods like French fries and potato chips
♦ skipping insulin to lose weight.

Parents are often shocked, baffled, and worried by this behavior. However, stay involved and interested in your teen's care. Your teen may be likely to take care of himself if he knows he is being supported and supervised.

If a teen and his parents are having a lot of problems related to diabetes care, an adult from outside the family (a coach, teacher, or nurse) may be able to provide the support the teen needs to manage his own care.

Setting realistic goals is important. If a teenager is only doing one blood test a day, negotiating with him to do two—and praising him when he does it—will be more successful than demanding he do four.

Sixteen-year-old Bob had a very busy schedule with school and sports and really couldn't do more than two blood tests a day. His mother scolded him for not doing more tests. At his most recent checkup he saw the diabetes educator, who said it was terrific that he did two blood tests a day. She didn't get upset or scold him. When she asked if Bob could try to do three tests on days when he played basketball, Bob thought he could handle that. With support and understanding, he had taken a step in the right direction.

Encouraging Independence

To help the teen with diabetes become independent, it is important to allow him to make decisions about his own care. Ideally, teens should already be making choices about meals and types and amounts of food. Remember, you're not going to be the one taking care of his diabetes when he's an adult—he is.

Let go gradually and allow the teen to take responsibility, as he feels ready, for blood testing and insulin injections. Your teen will make mistakes, but he will learn valuable lessons from them. You can help by making sure that proper supplies and foods are available.

Show that you are still interested and concerned about your teen by asking: "How are your tests running these days?" This shows that you expect your teen to be taking care of himself, but that you want to remain involved in his care.

Encourage your teen to develop a separate relationship with his doctor, dietitian, or diabetes educator. This can help him to find a treatment plan that he can live with. You can, of course, still talk to the doctor about concerns that you may have, but suggest that your teenager see his health care providers without you being present.

Try to be as loving, supportive, and patient as possible. It won't be easy, but many parents whose children don't have diabetes face similar problems. When the stresses of the teenage years seem to be creating great distress, psychological counseling may be helpful for teens and families. (See Asking for Help, page 186.) But most teens weather these stormy years quite well and become successful, self-assured adults.

Alcohol Use

Teenagers often want to try new and different things. Experimenting with alcohol is very common, even though it is illegal for teenagers to drink. Alcohol poses special risks for people with diabetes. Drinking alcohol can lower blood glucose, and the effect can occur hours afterwards. Combining alcohol with a sugary mixer or with too much food can raise blood glucose.

Alcohol can cloud judgment. A teen who has been drinking may forget his care plan or neglect to treat low blood glucose. He may think

Guidelines for Alcohol Use

Many adults with diabetes who drink moderately follow these guidelines.

- Know the harmful effects of alcohol. It's safest not to drink.
- Always wear your medical ID.
- Have no more than two drinks.
- Make sure that at least one person with you knows that you have diabetes and knows the signs of low blood glucose.
- Check your blood glucose from time to time. This is particularly important if you are doing anything physically active like dancing, playing ball, or swimming.
- Drink slowly. Sometimes one drink can satisfy a craving and allow you to feel part of the crowd.
- Know the alcohol content of various kinds of liquor. Light wines often have a low alcohol content. Dry wines often have less sugar than sweeter ones. Alcohol has no nutritional benefits. (For practical purposes, it is usually counted as a fat.)
- Alcohol may make you hungry, and you may forget the importance of sticking to your meal plan. When drinking, try to avoid bingeing on party snacks and desserts.
- If you have a mixed drink, avoid sugar-sweetened mixers. Mix alcohol with water, diet soda, or club soda to dilute it.
- Alcohol is safest when consumed as a part of a meal or scheduled snack. Don't substitute alcohol for meals or snacks and don't drink on an empty stomach.
- Drinking and driving is dangerous for everyone and is especially dangerous for people with diabetes. This is because alcohol may increase your risk of having a low blood glucose.
- If you are taking any medications such as antihistamines or cold remedies, talk to your health care provider about what effect they may have on alcohol or on your diabetes control.
- Check blood glucose levels at night (after drinking).

that alcohol is making him feel strange when the feeling may be partly caused by plummeting blood glucose levels. Other people may not notice the signs of low blood glucose and think, "He's just drunk." Or a profound low blood glucose can occur in the night.

Tobacco Use

Using tobacco in any form increases health risks. Smoking is linked to about 106,000 lung cancer deaths and about 225,000 heart disease deaths every year. Smoking can also cause high blood pressure, allergies, and ear and sinus infections.

People with diabetes already have a higher than average risk of getting heart disease, high blood pressure, and kidney disease. Combining smoking with diabetes further increases an individual's chances of having health problems.

Some teens chew tobacco or use snuff, thinking that these habits are less hazardous to health than smoking. In fact, the body absorbs more nicotine when tobacco is chewed or inhaled than when it is smoked. Chewing tobacco and snuff can make the nose and eyes run, cause irritation of the membranes in the nose and mouth, and lead to cancer of the nose and mouth.

In spite of these health risks, many teens choose to smoke or chew tobacco. Parents can help teens to decide against smoking by making the facts available—and by not smoking or chewing tobacco themselves.

When a person with diabetes tries to cut down on smoking or quit completely, he may experience symptoms of nicotine withdrawal (drowsiness, restless sleep, irritability, headache, and hunger) that are similar to symptoms of low blood glucose. Smoking cessation classes offered by high schools or community hospitals can be a source of support for those who are trying to give up tobacco use.

Illegal Drug Use

Some teens are attracted to illegal drugs like marijuana and cocaine. They may believe that these drugs are safe and that drug use is fun or a sign of maturity.

Before teens with diabetes consider using illegal drugs, they should know not only their general risks but also the special risks drugs pose to people with diabetes. Like alcohol, drugs can play havoc with blood glucose levels. In some case, drugs lower glucose levels and in other cases raise them. A person's response to a drug may mask the warning signs of low blood glucose.

Marijuana can make people very hungry. Eating too much can, of course, cause high blood glucose levels and weight gain. Marijuana use can also lead to an attitude of indifference, which affects the way a teen manages diabetes, and diabetes control can deteriorate.

It may be hard for parents to get this information across effectively. One approach may be to provide booklets about drug use that are written especially for teenagers and that suggest resources teenagers can turn to for help or additional information.

Try to keep the lines of communication open. Find a quiet moment to have a calm discussion about drugs with your teen and listen to what he has to say. You might tell him that you understand his curiosity about drugs and the pressure he may be under to try them. However, research has shown that teens who do not use drugs have made this decision partly because of parental influence. Their common response is "my parents would kill me!" So it is very important to stand firmly against drug use, and equally important to stay very aware of your child's activities and involved in his life.

Driving

Getting a driver's license is a big day in every teen's life. Driving should not be a problem for a teen with diabetes, but he will need a doctor's clearance and should always be prepared for hypoglycemia when driving.

Any driver with diabetes should always test his blood glucose before driving, unless he has just eaten. Your teen should always keep glucose gel or tablets, or packaged crackers in the glove compartment of his car. You never know when a traffic jam could delay a meal or snack! If your teen feels a low blood glucose episode coming on while driving, he should park the car right away, treat the low, and wait until his blood glucose level returns to normal.

Driving may be a problem for a person with diabetes who does not feel early warning signs of low blood glucose. Blood glucose testing before driving and at 2-hour intervals is essential for anyone who has

State Drivers' License Rules

All states have special licensing rules governing medical conditions that may apply to people with diabetes. Some states apply these rules to all drivers with diabetes, while many others apply them only to those who have actually experienced episodes of altered consciousness due to the disease or have other complications of diabetes. You can review your state's specific laws at www. diabetes.org/driving-with-diabetes/know-your-rights/discrimination/drivers-licenses/drivers-license-laws-by-state.html.

this problem. Continuous glucose monitoring can be very helpful in this situation as it will give a warning when blood glucoses are dropping. Wearing an ID tag is important in case of an accident.

Friends and Dating

Diabetes should not prevent a teen from having a full and fun-filled social life. For most teens, this will include dating. How to handle dating issues, however, is sometimes a concern. Teens have devised many successful approaches to handling diabetes while dating.

Your teen may wish to tell his girlfriend about diabetes. A brief explanation in advance may help him avoid alcohol or sweets at a party or clear the way for having a needed snack while out on a date. Explaining the signs of low blood glucose can help to prevent misunderstanding if your teen becomes irritable, pale, or restless.

Snacks should not be a problem on a date or at a party as long as they are included in his meal plan. Your teen can ask what food is being served at a party or discuss the choice of restaurant selections beforehand. Some teens bring their own sugar-free soft drinks to parties or their contribution to the food is a healthy choice that they can eat, such as cut fresh vegetables and dip. Most of the time, teens want parents to stay out of their food choices, and want to manage social events on their own. This is normal and acceptable, as long as they are doing a good job and making good choices. You child might need some opportunities to show you that she can be responsible in taking care of herself.

Eating Disorders

Eating disorders most often affect teenage girls and young women, but they can affect boys as well. A teen who is preoccupied with her weight or who feels she has no control over her life may be more likely to develop an eating disorder. Teenagers with diabetes may be at risk for eating disorders because they must focus on food and their meal plan. Because there are times when they must eat or drink, it may be harder for them to keep their weight under control. The two most common eating disorders in young women are:

♦ Anorexia nervosa. People lose weight by starving themselves.
♦ Bulimia. People sometimes starve themselves and sometimes go on food binges. After bingeing, they may make themselves throw up or take laxatives or water pills to purge the food and water. A teenager with diabetes who binges and then skips her insulin, wreaks havoc on her blood glucose levels and metabolism.

Your health care provider should be made aware of any eating disorders and should evaluate your teen, if necessary.

Common Signs of an Eating Disorder

A teenager who displays several of the following signs may have an eating disorder:

♦ extreme thinness
♦ wearing layers of clothes to cover what is perceived as fat
♦ cracks or redness in the corners of the mouth
♦ dark marks on the teeth, which indicate erosion of the enamel
♦ trips to the bathroom after meals or snacks
♦ preoccupation with food or exercise
♦ weight loss or decreased insulin dose without an explanation
♦ depression

Eating disorders can be life-threatening. If you suspect that your teenager is developing an eating disorder or skipping insulin, notify your health care provider right away.

Puberty and Sexual Development

Puberty produces many physical and hormonal changes as your child's body becomes that of an adult. Boys' bodies begin producing testosterone (male sex hormone), which causes muscle development, growth of facial and body hair, and deepening of the voice. In girls, estrogen (the female sex hormone) causes menstruation and the growth of breasts and pubic hair. These physical changes may be accompanied by emotional changes such as moodiness and irritability. Teens also usually begin to develop an interest in the opposite sex.

All children and teens grow and develop at different rates. Girls usually begin puberty at a younger age than boys do. Menstrual periods typically begin at age 12 to 13. However, heredity has a lot of influence on when your child reaches puberty.

Your son's growth and development will probably be similar to his father's and your daughter's will probably be similar to her mother's. For example, if Dad's voice changed at 15, Johnny's voice will probably change at around the same age. If Mom started having menstrual periods at 11, the chances are that Kerry will also start at that age.

If diabetes is well controlled it will not affect your child's growth and development. However, your health care provider should carefully monitor your child's height, weight, and physical development. The progress of pubertal development also has an effect on how much insulin your teen requires. Kids in the middle of puberty require a lot of insulin because their hormones are so active.

Teens with diabetes, like other teens, may be sexually active. It's essential to talk to your teen honestly and directly about the risks of sex. Teach him about the likelihood of contracting sexually transmitted diseases (STD) such as the HIV virus, herpes, and syphilis; the risk of pregnancy; and contraception. Send your teen the message that abstinence is the only certain way to avoid STDs and pregnancy.

Erectile dysfunction (the inability to have an erection) can occur in men who have had diabetes for many years. It is extremely rare among teenage boys with diabetes, but fear of it may be present even at an early age. Nerve damage caused by poor glucose control is one of the reasons men with diabetes develop erectile dysfunction. If your teenage son has concerns about this problem, a discussion with his doctor may help.

Yeast Infections

Girls with diabetes may get vaginal infections, especially if they have frequent high blood glucose levels. A fungus called Candida Albicans causes the most common vaginal infection, often called a yeast infection.

This fungus is normally present in the skin, mouth, intestinal tract, and vagina. When it multiplies abnormally, it can cause an infection. Having high blood glucose levels and taking antibiotics can cause an overgrowth of the fungus. Most of the time a yeast infection can be easily treated by improving blood glucose control and with an over-the-counter anti-fungal cream.

Symptoms of infection include itching, burning, and a thick, white or yellow vaginal discharge that can look like cottage cheese. These infections can usually be treated with over-the-counter suppositories or creams. Improving diabetes control can help prevent yeast infections.

Tips To Help Prevent Yeast Infections

Other ways girls with diabetes can protect themselves from Candida infections include:

♦ Drying the outside vaginal area thoroughly after a shower, bath, or swim. Yeast is less likely to grow in a dry area.

♦ Wiping from front to back after going to the bathroom.

♦ Changing out of a wet bathing suit or other wet clothes quickly.

♦ Wearing cotton underwear.

♦ Avoiding wearing nylon (nonbreathing) clothing, such as spandex tights or shorts, for long periods of time.

♦ Avoiding wearing extremely tight jeans.

♦ Babies with diabetes can also develop rashes at their diaper area when glucose is high in their urine. If the child is not potty trained and blood glucose is high, careful attention to the diaper area and frequent changing is important.

Marriage

Teenagers with diabetes may have concerns about marriage. There are all kinds of questions that crop up when there is a chronic illness such as diabetes, and of course, there are considerations that must be made to accommodate meal plans, eating habits, and healthy lifestyle.

The partner of a person with diabetes may face some lifestyle changes. He must understand his partner's need to take insulin, to stick to a meal plan, and to check blood glucose levels frequently. The partner may have to deal with mood swings that can occur with changes in blood glucose levels, or beeping pumps in the night. Some partners may feel anxious about treating low blood glucose episodes. In many cases, partners can benefit from attending diabetes education classes.

Pregnancy

Diabetes need not prevent most women from having a family. Pregnancy does pose extra risks to both the woman with diabetes and her baby, but with good medical care a woman with diabetes can give birth to a healthy infant. The most important thing she needs to do is to work toward optimal diabetes control (normal numbers) prior to becoming pregnant, and try her best to sustain normal blood sugars through-out the pregnancy. Achieving good diabetes control before becoming pregnant is extremely important.

"Of 100 children born to a parent with type I diabetes, between I and 8 children may get diabetes."

Uncontrolled diabetes during the first few weeks of pregnancy can cause birth defects. Prenatal care and tight control of blood glucose levels during pregnancy help to assure the birth of a healthy baby. If your health care provider has not spoken to your teen daughter about the risks of unplanned pregnancy, it is important that you do or request that they do.

Teenagers may wonder whether their children will also get diabetes. Research shows that some people do inherit a higher risk of getting diabetes. Recent studies show that of 100 children born to a parent with type 1 diabetes, between 1 and 8 may get diabetes. A couple in which one partner has diabetes may wish to get genetic counseling before starting a family.

Career Choices

Many teenagers wonder, "Will diabetes limit my career choices?" The most honest answer to this question is "yes and no." By law, a person with type 1 diabetes cannot enlist in the military or pilot a commercial aircraft. With these exceptions, however, most occupations are open to people with diabetes.

Some laws excluding people with diabetes from certain types of work have been successfully challenged. For example, at one time people with diabetes could not drive commercial vehicles such as trucks or buses. Now, however, people with diabetes may be accepted as truck or bus drivers on a case-by-case basis.

People with diabetes are protected against job discrimination by many state and federal laws. A person who feels that he has been discriminated against may contact the American Diabetes Association at www.diabetes.org for further information about these laws and the possible recourse against discrimination.

Advances in the treatment of diabetes have opened professional doors. People with diabetes are working in many careers, including police work and fire fighting. Like all people, teens with diabetes should choose careers based on their talents, interests, and qualifications.

This being said, people with diabetes have been able to tackle careers in professional sports, politics, acting, music, the media, medicine, and the list goes on and on. The box on the next page is just a short small number of the well-known celebrities and athletes that have diabetes.

Famous People With Diabetes

People with diabetes are among the leading doctors, scientists, political leaders, teachers, and lawyers in the U.S. A few of the celebrities and sports figures with diabetes in the U.S. are:

Halle Berry (actress)

Mary Tyler Moore (actress)

Morgan Freeman (actor)

Randy Jackson (host of American Idol, music producer)

Salma Hayek (actress)

Larry King (media personality)

Ray Kroc (McDonald's founder)

Sonia Sotomayor (Supreme Court Justice)

Bret Michaels (musician)

Tony Bennett (musician)

Nick Jonas (musician, Jonas Brothers)

Aretha Franklin (musician)

B.B. King (musician)

Jay Cutler (NFL football)

Kelli Kuehne (LPGA golf)

Adam Morrison (NBA basketball)

Chapter 9:
Living with Diabetes

L iving successfully with diabetes isn't always easy, but with discipline, patience, and good medical care, it can be done. Everything about life with diabetes is a balancing act. You have to balance food, insulin, and activity to keep blood glucose levels within a target range. Your child with diabetes depends on you for care and support. He will follow your lead. If you can feel comfortable and positive about your child's condition, he will learn to feel the same way. If you have a can-do attitude when faced with life's surprises, he'll take on challenges with the same outlook.

When your child is very young, you will do all of the day-to-day tasks of caring for his diabetes. As your child grows up, it's important that he gradually learns to take on these tasks for himself. It's important that you stay involved in your child's care even as you let your child take on more responsibility. This, too, is a balancing act.

The child who learns to live with diabetes has to do many things that other children don't have to do and make many decisions that other children don't have to make. He learns early in life the importance of being disciplined and taking responsibility for himself. These are lessons that can prepare your child for life as an adult. Learning to live successfully with diabetes can, ultimately, be an experience that enriches your child's whole life.

BUDGETING

Your dietitian can give you some useful hints about how to prepare inexpensive, healthful meals for your entire family. As with food, when shopping for diabetes supplies, it helps to compare prices, use coupons, and buy in bulk.

Always compare prices of supplies before buying. Companies that offer mail order diabetes supplies will vary in price, selection, and service. It pays to shop around.

TRAVELING

Vacations and trips are special times. A trip means a break from school, work, and the everyday routine. Unfortunately, it doesn't mean a break from diabetes care. Diabetes never takes a vacation, so it's best to always be prepared for the unexpected.

If your child is taking a long trip, it's a good idea for her to have a complete medical checkup before leaving. Take a record of the checkup along on the trip in case of hospitalization, injury, or other emergency. Important information in the record should include insulin dose and blood test results.

When making flight reservations, check the times that meals and snacks will be served. It's a good idea to bring extra food like crackers or fruit so your child can stay on schedule.

If you are traveling to a different time zone, get advice from your health care provider about how to adjust the timing of meals, insulin injections, and so on.

Packing

Pack diabetes supplies so they are always within easy reach. When traveling by plane, take syringes and insulin in a carry-on bag. This protects you in case your luggage is lost.

Insulin need not be packed in a thermos or ice chest. But insulin bottles should be kept in a cool, dry place and protected from breakage. Insulin should not be exposed to extreme heat or cold, so don't pack it in the trunk of a hot car or keep it in the glove compartment.

Always carry an emergency kit for hypoglycemia (low blood glucose) with you when traveling (see Your Emergency Kit, next page). Pack extra food, syringes, and insulin in a second bag in case one becomes lost.

Your child should wear a medical ID tag (see Should My Child

Your Emergency Kit

- a rapid-acting sugar (such as fruit juice or glucose tablets)
- a long-acting carbohydrate and protein (such as peanut butter or cheese crackers or nuts)
- a glucagon kit

Wear a Medical ID Tag?, page 114). The packet should include your physician's name and phone number and spare prescriptions for insulin, syringes, and glucagon.

Carry a physician-signed statement of your diabetes when you are traveling. You should have a letter of medical necessity that states that your child has diabetes and it is medically necessary that you carry all diabetes supplies including lancets, syringes, insulin, snacks, glucagon, and insulin pump.

Dealing with Emergencies

If you are traveling to a foreign country where most people don't speak English, it is helpful to learn some key phrases in the local language:

- "My child has diabetes" or "I have diabetes."
- "The child needs (I need) food/juice/sugar."
- "Please call a doctor."

Your child's doctor may be able to give you the name of an English-speaking doctor or hospital in the country you are visiting. In an emergency, the U.S. Embassy may be able to help.

SOLVING DAY-TO-DAY CHALLENGES

Many times parents ask for advice on specific childhood challenges that crop up with diabetes. Two main areas of difficulty seem to exist for parents: helping their children deal with their feelings about having diabetes, and getting their kids to cooperate with diabetes care routines.

Dealing With Feelings

Many people will try to reassure you when you find out your child has diabetes. They will tell you that your child has every chance of living a full, normal life with diabetes. Although these statements are generally true, they do not have a reassuring ring to them. Having diabetes is not normal, and testing blood and giving injections is not a normal activity for children and teens. Having diabetes is not easy, and having angry or sad feelings about it is to be expected.

Dealing with your child's feelings can be difficult and painful. But having your child talk about feelings is important, especially with you. There are certain skills parents can use to encourage conversations about feelings with their children. To keep the communication going:

- ♦ listen with your full attention
- ♦ accept your child's feelings without denying them
- ♦ acknowledge with one word.

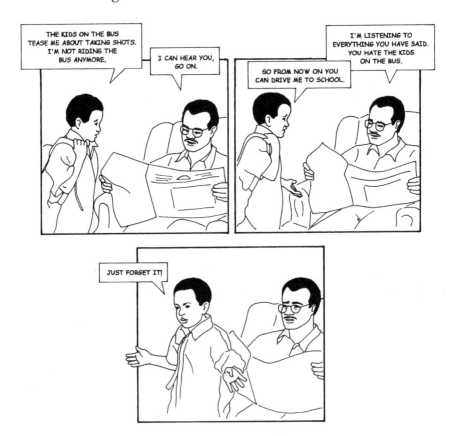

Listen with your full attention

Many parents with busy schedules (especially when diabetes care is added in) do not find it easy to stop what they are doing to listen to their children. It is discouraging for a child to try to get through to someone who is only half-listening. It is much more rewarding to tell your troubles to a parent who is really listening.

Careful listening is hard work. Many times parents are waiting for their children to finish talking so they can say what they want to say. Although it does require effort at the time, the time spent listening to your child will pay off.

If your child comes to you with a concern, stop what you are doing, sit down, and listen. Sometimes, a parent doesn't need to say anything. Often an understanding silence is all the child needs to solve her own problems.

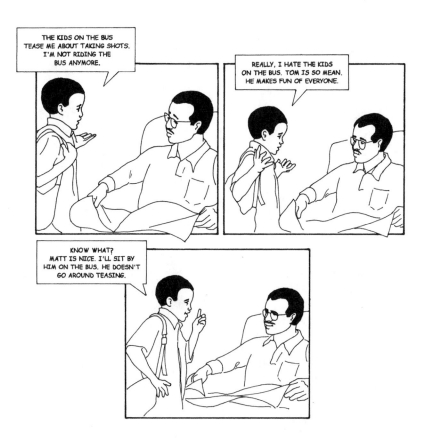

Accept your child's feelings without denying them

Try not to deny what your child is feeling. Sometimes parents feel so badly about the diabetes, they try to help their children by making diabetes seem like a smaller problem than it really is. In other words, parents are denying the way the child really feels. Saying things like, "You can handle it, there's no need to be upset," "It doesn't hurt that much!" and "It's not so bad" tell your child her feelings are not valid.

It's often easier for parents to understand how denying feelings affects communication when they put themselves in their child's place. For example, imagine if you were told to lose weight and needed to cut out desserts. You really enjoy desserts, and you share your frustration with a friend. Your friend responds by saying, "That's no big deal!"

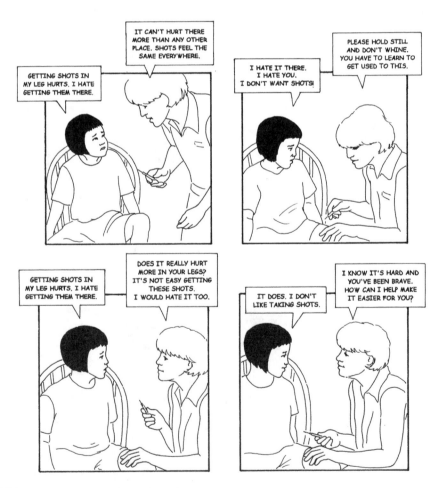

and "It's easy to avoid sweets." How would you feel?

You might feel angry that your friend doesn't understand. You may think there is no point in talking to this friend again about your frustration. Wouldn't it have been easier to talk to your friend if she accepted your feelings? What if she had said, "It must be tough for you. I like desserts too. I would hate missing them."

Try to tune in to your child's true feelings, and helpful words will often come to you. For example, you may find yourself saying, "Wow! You must still be hungry, even though you just had lunch," or "I can see that this shot hurt a little more than usual."

Remember that you and your child are separate people, and feel very differently about things. Acknowledge your child's separate reality.

Acknowledge with one word

Instead of asking a lot of questions and giving advice, sometimes it is better to acknowledge your child's feelings with just a word. Children, especially teens, don't always appreciate questions or advice. It is hard for a child to think clearly about a problem if someone is blaming, criticizing, or giving advice. Phrases like "You know what I think you should do?" or "If you're smart you'll always carry glucose tablets with you, so nothing like this happens again," or "I keep telling you to keep your meter in the nurse's office. You lost it before!" are not helpful.

> "There's a lot to be gained when parents allow their children to solve their own problems."

To get your child to continue talking about her feelings, sometimes it is helpful for a parent to simply say "Oh" or "Hmmm" or "I see." Words like these often open the door for your child to continue exploring his own thoughts.

There's a lot to be gained when parents allow their children to solve their own problems by encouraging them with simple words. Words like these combined with a caring, listening approach are invitations for children to explore their own thoughts and find their own solutions.

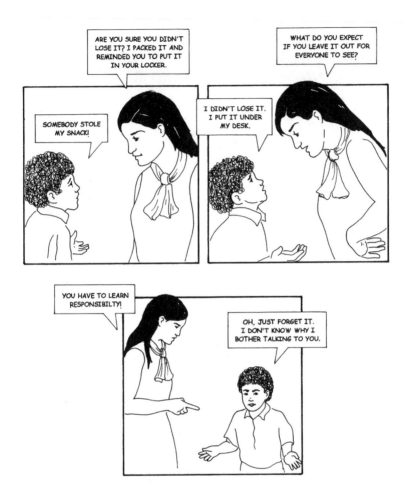

Getting Cooperation

One of the toughest jobs for a parent is trying to get children to do what they are supposed to do. The daily struggles of getting children to make their beds, brush their teeth, do homework, or walk the dog are quite enough. With diabetes there are even more struggles: doing the blood tests, carrying snacks, giving injections, and so on.

Parents often complain that they feel like nags. Children often say their parents are slave drivers who have an endless stream of tedious tasks for them to do. Most parents have heard the words. "You just don't understand!" That is a true statement! In most cases, parents, really do not have a grasp on what their children must deal with.

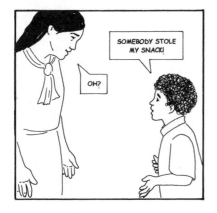
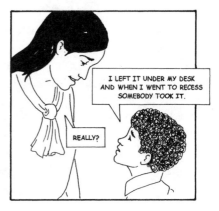
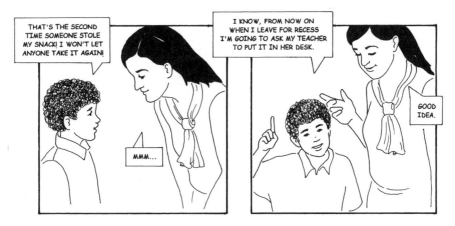

Some parents blame or accuse: "How many times do I have to tell you to wash your hands before testing?" "You never wear your ID bracelet. I paid good money for that!" "The trouble with you is you never tell the doctor the truth!"

Some parents give commands: "I want you to record your blood sugar right now!" "Hurry up and take your shot—the bus is coming!"

Some use warnings: "You better be careful or you'll end up in the hospital." "You better not do that again or you will go low."

And other parents are martyrs: "I'm drained from dealing with all of this and you don't make it any easier." "Are you trying to give me a heart attack?"

♦ Describe what you see or describe the problem. Don't accuse. It's easier to think about the problem when someone explains it to you.

♦ Use fewer words.

♦ Listen to their feelings and express your own feelings.

♦ Write a note to remind them to take their insulin, eat a snack before practice, etc.

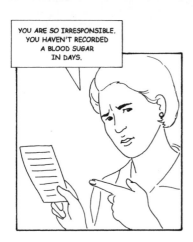

YOU ARE SO IRRESPONSIBLE. YOU HAVEN'T RECORDED A BLOOD SUGAR IN DAYS.

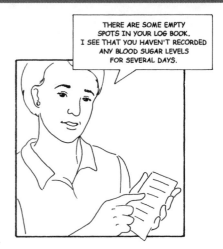

THERE ARE SOME EMPTY SPOTS IN YOUR LOG BOOK. I SEE THAT YOU HAVEN'T RECORDED ANY BLOOD SUGAR LEVELS FOR SEVERAL DAYS.

Sharing Thoughts

Here are some thoughts that your teen most likely would like you to understand about how she feels about having diabetes.

Your teen wants you to appreciate that it is difficult to have diabetes, yet doesn't want you to be too sympathetic. She wants you to know that the biggest thing is that she doesn't want to feel different from her friends. She doesn't like having to test her blood sugar in front of everyone; yet, doesn't like to have to leave her friends to test her blood. She misses having freedom to eat what she pleases. She finds it rude when people presume she can't eat things she actually can have, so they don't even offer it to her. She says that it doesn't bother her when others eat

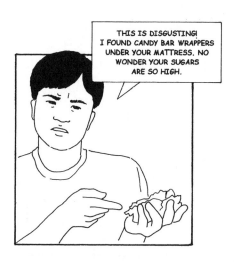
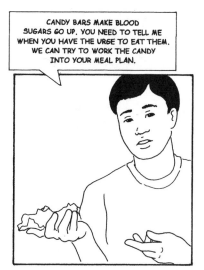

candy and desserts in front of her, but it does bother her. She wonders if her best friend really cares about her when she encourages her to eat candy and other things she shouldn't be eating. She feels that she is expected not to want something she does want. When her siblings eat ice cream, sometimes her discipline crumbles and she eats too much. But she also worries that her siblings will resent her because they are not allowed to have candy and brownies in the house because of her diabetes.

If she is overweight, she wants you to know how depressing it feels to be heavier than her friends, and sometimes ridiculed by her peers for being so. She wants to diet, but if she tries on her own, will usually be hypoglycemic. She wants to hear from you that if she works hard to follow her meal plan that she can lose the weight and be healthy. She wants you to believe in her and help her with it. She does not want to hear negative things about being overweight.

In spite of all her failures, she wants you to know that the most important thing to her is the love and approval of you, her parents. Most of the time she has trouble expressing it, but she ultimately desires a close relationship. She wants encouragement and role modeling from you on how to eat right and exercise. The discipline you show in your life sets an example for her to follow.

Your teen also prefers that you allow him to handle his diabetes in his own way, as long as he is being responsible in caring for himself. He

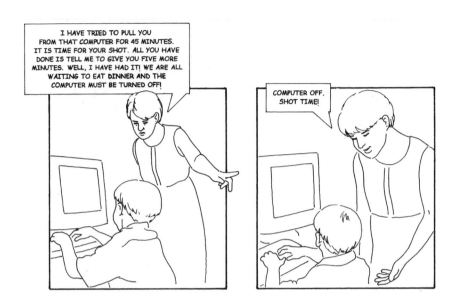

is growing up, turning in to a man, and needs to learn to take care of himself. He may want to tell friends and others about diabetes himself, or not. He probably will want you to withhold announcements about "holding the sauce because he has diabetes" to others, such as to the waitress and others seated at the table. There may be instances where he'd like you to ease his way by helping him tell others. He'll tell you when these times are, but most of the time he'd prefer to tell others himself.

He gets furious when you remind him to test his blood sugar or record the number in a log, yet cannot seem to remember to do it himself. He doesn't want you to be involved in his diabetes care because he wants to be independent. He wants to do it himself and wants you to know that you can trust him, yet he can't seem to always follow through. He knows that sometimes he slips up on his testing, or eats extra food, but doesn't want you to be worried or angry with him when he has high numbers. Sometimes he knows why his numbers are high (because he ate too much) and sometimes he has no idea why his blood sugar numbers are high. When you get upset, worried, or "freak out" when numbers are high, he resorts to keeping the peace by giving you the numbers that you want to see. He'd like to be honest about it, but doesn't want to worry you any more than he already has. And he doesn't want more nagging than he already receives.

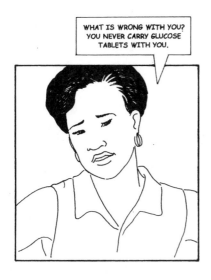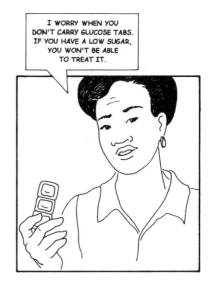

Frequently, other things get in the way of the things he intends to do. In spite of the fact that he pushes you away, he really relies on your power and protection. He needs to know that you will protect him from himself, if need be. He needs to know that you care and will be involved in his care, no matter what he says and does. He actually feels very scared when he thinks about being completely at the mercy of his own self-control and self-discipline.

She also wants you to understand what an enormous inconvenience it is. She now has to take insulin wherever she goes, in case she'd be out for dinner. Although most of her friends are supportive, she doesn't like the attention she gets. She doesn't like the bruising in her arms and legs, or puffy spots in her tummy. She doesn't like to feel low and have to eat glucose tablets in the middle of class with everybody watching her. Neither does she like to have to leave class and go to the nurse's office. She is embarrassed when others fuss over her when she is feeling symptoms of hypoglycemia.

Your teen wants you to know that the responsibility of diabetes has taken some of the joy and spontaneity out of her life. She now has to be prepared for any occurrence, and travel with equipment and medication. It is a bit frightening, and she tries not to think of all the bad things that could happen. She had never before thought of being sick or dying, and now she has a disease that suggests she could have frightening complications unless she follows her program. She's doing the best she can, and doesn't want to be sick now or in the future. She wonders how she is supposed to balance all the things that are important to her—friends, school, activities—AND keep diabetes a top priority.

WHEN PARENTS ARE SINGLE OR DIVORCED

As the media frequently reminds us, today's culture and society has a staggering number of single parents and a divorce rate of about 50%. Single parents struggle to do all that is expected and required, and when their child has diabetes, it can become an overwhelming and relentless effort for one person to take on. And when parents divorce, it brings momentous change and raises difficult issues for the whole family. Even in the best of circumstances, when separated parents remain amicable, cooperative, and willing to communicate, divorce can cause emotional distress, create financial difficulties, and bring about major life changes, such as moving into a new home, attending a new school, finding a new job, or perhaps reentering the workforce.

When there is tension within a family, a child's diabetes may take a backseat to more urgent issues, or it may become a focal point of contention and strife. Often, a child in this situation feels stress (perhaps because he thinks he must smooth things out between his parents), which can cause high blood glucose. In other cases, divorce can actually be an improvement for the child, due to the establishment of a more peaceful and stable home environment.

Both parents and the children will need time to grieve the breakup of the family and may struggle with feelings of guilt, sadness, anger, loneliness, anxiety, shame, and even depression. For divorced parents of a child with diabetes, dealing with these feelings and learning to communicate and share parental responsibilities is crucial to protect the emotional health of the child and ensure that his diabetes is well controlled.

After parents separate, it often becomes apparent that lifestyles are very different. Eating and sleeping schedules, quality and quantity of foods, parental oversight and permissiveness, activities, and diabetes supervision might be noticeably different. When parents have widely differing approaches to diabetes management, the child may feel insecure. He might be afraid that his diabetes is not being treated properly by one or both parents, or he may be confused about the importance of managing it at all. Sometimes, children have expressed that they think the more permissive parent doesn't care as much. Either way, each parent must take responsibility for learning as much as possible about the subtleties and daily management of their child's diabetes, so that both have equal skill in managing it. Accepting responsibility for your child's care means being willing to work together with your former spouse so that your child will feel safe and have better diabetes control.

Good communication between parents involves clearly expressing expectations and sharing necessary medical information, including contact information for the child's health care team. Every time the child visits the other parent or switches homes for a while, the following information should be exchanged:

♦ General information about how the child has been feeling lately. Discuss your child's average and out-of-range blood glucose levels, any episodes of hypoglycemia or presence of ketones in the urine, a cold, fever, or other illness that might affect his blood glucose control and meal plan, and any changes in insulin doses.

♦ Specific information about that day. Explain when and what the child last ate, how much insulin he's taken or exercise he's had that day, and when and what his last several blood glucose readings were. Writing this information down and transferring a copy of recent blood glucose results and insulin doses is helpful if talk is strained and in case of a medical emergency.

♦ Any difficulties that occurred after the last visit. The intention here is not to lay blame but to provide information. Dad may not realize that Johnny's blood sugar is over 300 mg/dl every Sunday night after he brings him back to his mother. If he knows this, he can make insulin or meal plan adjustments so that Johnny can enjoy his Sunday night Dairy Queen treat without high blood glucose later on.

Sometimes the effects of different schedules on the child's blood glucose levels are obvious, and other times they are not. One trick that can help make things clear is to maintain a monthly rather than weekly record of blood glucose readings and to mark out-of-range blood glucose numbers with different colored highlighters.

Sometimes it becomes clear that Tommy's blood sugar is always lower at Dad's because he is more active there, and higher at Mom's because meals are larger. That does not mean one lifestyle is right and one is wrong, just that they are different. Therefore, it is quite important to figure it out because Tommy might need less insulin on the days he is at Dad's than the days he is at Mom's. A diabetes educator or your doctor will be able to assist you in making these adjustments.

A child's diagnosis of diabetes creates lifelong parental challenges that you may just be beginning to encounter. If separated parents are able to come together on diabetes care, they can give their child a valuable lesson in handling this and other life changes in a healthy manner. Try to stay focused and be persistent in your efforts; your child deserves nothing less.

COPING WITH DIABETES

Having a child with diabetes can be very stressful for you and your family. It can be hard to accept that your child has a disease that isn't going to go away and that needs care and attention every day. Caring for a child with diabetes alters your family routine and can affect relationships among family members.

Having diabetes is stressful for your child, too. Young children may think that diabetes is a punishment for something they did. It's important to try to reassure your child that having diabetes isn't her fault.

Feeling loved by the whole family can help your child to accept having diabetes. Involving everyone in the family in your child's care can help to make diabetes a normal part of family life.

Parents often worry about disciplining a child with diabetes because it can be hard to tell the difference between normal misbehavior and signs of low blood glucose. It's important, however, not to treat your child with diabetes differently from your other children. Ordinary discipline should not have any effect on your child's blood glucose level.

Important Tips for Parents

♦ When it is time to make a decision about an activity, ask yourself what you would or wouldn't allow your child to do if they did not have diabetes. If your child is being responsible in his diabetes care, and you would otherwise allow the activity, give him a chance to prove his ability to care for himself.

♦ Kids who do well with their care generally have a parent, or sometimes a grandparent, who stays involved in the diabetes care and keeps the kid accountable. This person is the organizer and the person who will check the numbers in the meter memory to make sure tests are being done.

♦ Understand that when it comes to doing diabetes tasks, there is not a steady progression from one stage to the next as teens mature. They ebb and flow in their ability and capability to take care of themselves. Periodically, you may need to step in and take over a task that your child had previously been doing. This effort is usually temporary, as he regroups and begins to move forward again.

♦ Don't assume that your child or teen is following his diabetes program. Countless parents are surprised when meters or pumps are uploaded at the doctor's office and they find their child has not been doing what they are supposed to be doing. Stay tuned in to what they are doing.

♦ Kids learn how to cope and behave from their parents. Therefore, it is important for you as a parent to model the ways you would like your children to behave. Set a good example. If you take care of yourself, eat well, exercise, and establish good sleep habits, it is very likely that your children will as well.

♦ Don't hesitate to seek professional counseling for yourself, your child, or your family. It is hard enough to grow up these days without the additional burden of diabetes.

ASKING FOR HELP

Every family will go through times when it's hard to cope with the demands of diabetes on top of the stresses of everyday life. During these difficult periods, you and your family may benefit from the help of a professional counselor.

Professional counselors are trained to help people with special problems and concerns. Many people are ashamed to ask for this kind of help. Some think that asking for help makes them a failure. Others fear being labeled mentally ill. These concerns are understandable, but unjustified. There is no shame in asking for help. Caring for a child with diabetes is a hard job. Knowing when you need extra help is a sign of mental health, not mental illness. Counseling can make a real difference in how diabetes affects you and your child. Many families find that just one session with a counselor makes a big difference.

> "There is no shame in asking for help. Caring for a child with diabetes is a hard job."

How do you find a counselor that you like and feel comfortable with? If a health care team cares for your child, the team may include a counselor (a social worker, psychologist, or psychiatrist). Your child's doctor may be able to refer you to a good counselor. Many communities have family service organizations that offer counseling.

You may want to go to a meeting of a support group affiliated with the American Diabetes Association. These groups usually meet informally. They offer a chance for your child to meet other children with diabetes and for you to meet other parents of children with diabetes. Parents can exchange experiences, problems, and solutions. Families can see that they are not alone and that other families are facing similar challenges.

Look at www.diabetes.org to see if there is an American Diabetes Association chapter in your area. The American Diabetes Association also has many books, pamphlets, and other publications about diabetes available (see Resources, page 201).

TRANSITIONING TO ADULT CARE

Children who have grown up under the umbrella of pediatric care often have difficulty moving to adult care; however, those who have formed positive habits throughout their teen years generally do well when they start to manage their diabetes on their own. The time between finishing high school and moving into the adult world can be a tough one because of all the changes your child will experience. Luckily, new legislation will help to provide medical coverage for these young adults who are not in school. This is helpful as teenagers may need to start all over with diabetes education in order to care for themselves without constant parental support.

One of the most important things to remember is that they continue to be seen by a physician every 3 months. Those who do not follow through are at greater risk for complications of diabetes. It is a scary time for parents who are caught in the conflict of hanging on/letting go. In general, those children who have had good support growing up have formed positive habits and are more than capable of handling their own care. Some pediatric diabetes programs even have formal education for parents and teens about what to expect as teens move toward adult care. Check with your health care provider.

Appendix

The next few pages give instructions on how to draw up single or multiple types of insulin. There are also instructions on where to give insulin injections. Find more information on types of insulin and other methods of administering insulin in Chapter 3, page 25.

Where To Give Injections

Where to give injections in your child's arm:

- ♦ Ask your child to put her left hand on her right arm (by the shoulder) with her fingers closed. The bottom of the hand is the highest point where injections should be given.
- ♦ Next, ask your child to grab her arm just above the right elbow. The top of the hand is the lowest point where injections should be given.
- ♦ In the space between your child's hands, draw two imaginary lines down the arm—one down the side and one down the middle of the back of the arm.
- ♦ Give the injections along these two tracks, measuring from one spot to the next by the width of two of your child's fingers.

Where to give injections in your child's abdomen:

- ♦ Draw an imaginary one-inch circle around your child's navel. Don't give injections inside the circle because this area can be tender.
- ♦ Give the injections in the surrounding area of the abdomen, stomach, and hip.

(continued)

Where to give injections in your child's thigh:

♦ Ask your child to put one hand at the top of her thigh (by the hip) and the other hand on top of her knee on the same leg. It's okay to give injections in the space between the hands.

♦ Draw three imaginary lines, one down the top of the leg and one on each side—one toward the outside and one toward the inside.

♦ Give the injections along these three tracks, measuring from one spot to the next by the width of two of your child's fingers.

♦ Another good spot in a child with muscular thighs is the traditional "saddle-bag" area (the upper outer thigh).

Where to give injections in your child's hip:

♦ The upper outer quadrant of the buttock (actually the hip) is a suitable place for injections, although it may be a difficult area for your child to reach to give her own injections. Check with your child's doctor for instructions on giving injections in the hip.

If your child gets puffiness or lumps near the area of an injection:

♦ Don't give any more injections in that spot for 3–6 months. The lumps should go away eventually.

How To Draw Up One Type of Insulin

1. Wash your hands.
2. Select the injection site according to your rotation schedule (see What Is Site Rotation?, on page 35).
3. Clean the injection site with soap and water or alcohol. (Alcohol may be used, but it dries the skin.)
4. If you are using a cloudy insulin, such as NPH, gently roll the insulin bottle between your hands to mix the insulin. Wipe the top of the insulin bottle with alcohol.
5. Draw back the plunger on the syringe to the correct number of insulin units.
6. Holding the insulin bottle upright, insert the needle into the bottle and push the plunger in. This injects air into the bottle.
7. Keeping the needle in the bottle, turn the bottle upside down and slowly pull back the plunger until the syringe has more insulin in it than you need.
8. Gently tap the syringe to move air bubbles to the top.
9. With the needle still in the bottle, slowly press the plunger forward to expel the air bubbles and extra insulin.
10. Double-check that you have the correct number of insulin units in the syringe.
11. Gently pull the needle out of the bottle.

How To Draw Up Two Types of Insulin

1. Wash your hands thoroughly.
2. Select the injection site according to your rotation schedule (see What Is Site Rotation?, on page 35).
3. Clean the injection site with soap and water or alcohol. (Alcohol may be used if it is more convenient, but it dries the skin.)
4. Gently roll the cloudy (intermediate-acting) insulin bottle between your hands to mix the insulin. Wipe the top of the insulin bottles with alcohol.
5. Draw back the plunger on the syringe to the correct number of units of cloudy insulin to be given.
6. Holding the bottle of cloudy insulin upright, insert the needle into the bottle and push the plunger in. This injects air into the bottle.
7. Keeping the needle in the bottle, turn the bottle of cloudy insulin upside down and slowly pull back the plunger until the syringe has more insulin in it than you need.
8. Gently tap the syringe to move air bubbles to the top.
9. With the needle still in the bottle, slowly press the plunger forward to expel the air bubbles and extra insulin.
10. Double-check that you have the correct number of units of cloudy (intermediate-acting) insulin in the syringe.
11. Gently pull the needle out of the bottle.
12. Draw back the plunger on the syringe to the correct number of units of clear (short-acting) insulin to be given.
    13. Holding the bottle of clear (short-acting) insulin upright, insert the needle into the air space in the bottle and push the plunger in. This injects air into the bottle. Remove the needle.

(continued)

14. Insert the needle into the bottle of clear (short-acting) insulin and slowly withdraw the correct number of units. Take care that none of the insulin already in the syringe is pushed into the bottle of rapid-acting insulin. If the insulins are accidentally mixed in the bottle, you must discard the bottle of rapid-acting insulin because it may not act quickly anymore.

15. Check for air bubbles in the syringe. If there is a large air bubble in the syringe after you have added the short-acting insulin, discard the syringe and start again. If there is a small air bubble that can be tapped out without noticeably changing the dosage, go ahead and give the injection. Small air bubbles will not harm your child, but they can alter the amount of insulin injected.

Glossary

A1C: A test that shows a person's average blood glucose level over a period of 2–3 months, usually shown as a percentage. The A1C test measures the amount of gylcosylated hemoglobin in the blood.

Adrenaline: A hormone that helps the body deal with stress. By making the body produce more glucose, adrenaline can raise the blood glucose level.

Antibody: A protein, made in response to a bacteria or virus, that fights infection.

Autoimmune disorder: A disease in which antibodies, instead of helping the body fight infection, attack normal parts of the body. For example, antibodies may attack and destroy the cells that make insulin, causing diabetes.

Beta cells: Small clumps of cells in the pancreas that make insulin. In type 1 diabetes, these cells are destroyed and no longer can produce insulin.

Carbohydrate: The body's preferred source of energy. There are two kinds of carbohydrates: simple sugars, which the body processes quickly, and complex carbohydrates, which generally take more time to digest. Simple sugars cause a rapid rise in the blood glucose level. Complex carbohydrates tend to cause a more gradual rise in blood glucose.

Cardiovascular: Relating to the heart and blood vessels.

Cell: The basic structural unit of all animals and plants. Cells are the physical basis of all life processes.

Cell membrane: Material that surrounds each cell. The membrane keeps in substances that the cell needs and excludes harmful ones.

Choices/Exchange: One way of planning food that was more popular in the past. Basically, one "exchange" is a portion size based on carbohydrates, proteins, fat, and calories in one portion. Exchange Lists divide food into six categories: starch, meat, vegetable, fruit, milk, and fat. Each list consists of foods that, in the stated amounts, can be "exchanged" or substituted for any other food on the same list.

Diabetes educator: A health care professional who has specialized training in the care of diabetes. A diabetes educator may be a nurse, a dietitian, a pharmacist, a social worker, a physician, or may be trained in another health care field. A Certified Diabetes Educator (CDE) has passed a qualifying exam and has spent a specific amount of time teaching people about diabetes.

Dietitian: A health care professional who has specialized training in diet and nutrition. A Registered Dietitian (RD) has passed a qualifying exam.

Endocrinologist: A physician who specializes in the treatment of diseases caused by imbalances of hormones. Diabetes is one such disease. Some endocrinologists who specialize in treating patients with diabetes call themselves diabetologists.

Estimated Average Glucose (eAG): A new way to report A1C numbers that interpret your A1C as an average glucose number. It is often easier to understand because it is reported in mg/dl, just like when you take your blood glucose on a meter.

Fats: A food group and a source of energy for the body. Fats do not raise blood glucose very much, but some kinds of fat raise the cholesterol level in the blood.

Gingivitis: Inflammation of the gums. Gingivitis can be a long-term complication of diabetes, but it can be reduced or prevented with regular dental care.

Glucagon: A hormone produced in the pancreas. Glucagon raises blood glucose levels. It is also given by injection for treating very low blood glucose if a person cannot eat or drink or is unconscious.

Glucose: A kind of carbohydrate, glucose is the body's main source of energy. The digestive system makes glucose by breaking down carbohydrate.

Glycemic response: The rate and amount by which a certain food raises blood glucose.

Glycosuria: Glucose in the urine.

Hormone: A substance made by an endocrine gland that aids growth or body functioning. Adrenaline, glucagon, and insulin are hormones.

Hyperglycemia: A high level of glucose in the blood. Common symptoms include frequent urination, excessive thirst, weight loss, increased appetite, tiredness, and blurred vision. Hyperglycemia is a sign of uncontrolled diabetes. It may be treated by giving a bigger dose of insulin or by getting exercise to lower blood glucose levels. Untreated, hyperglycemia can lead to ketoacidosis.

Hyperlipidemia: A high level of fats in the blood.

Hypoglycemia: A low level of glucose in the blood. Common symptoms include nervousness, headache, pallor, fatigue, weakness, nightmares, hunger, irritability, sweating, personality changes, shakiness, and confusion. Hypoglycemia must be treated quickly. Untreated, it can lead to seizures and unconsciousness. Treat hypoglycemia with carbohydrates to raise blood glucose levels quickly.

Insulin: A hormone made in the beta cells of the pancreas. It allows the body to use glucose for energy.

Insulin resistance: A condition common in type 2 diabetes, where the body is unable to use circulating insulin.

Islets of Langerhans: Clusters of cells in the pancreas. The islets are made of four kinds of cells. Beta cells are the ones that make insulin.

Juvenile-onset diabetes: Former name for type 1 diabetes, also previously called "insulin dependent diabetes mellitus."

Ketoacidosis: A serious condition that demands attention. Ketones, byproducts of fat digestion, build up in the body, creating acidity in the blood. Symptoms include nausea, vomiting, fruity-smelling breath, dry skin, labored breathing, and stupor, which can lead to diabetic coma. Usually occurs at diagnosis of diabetes, or with flu or illness.

Ketone: A waste product made by the body when it burns fat for energy.

Ketonemia: Ketones in the blood.

Ketonuria: Ketones in the urine.

Kidney: One of a pair of organs that functions to remove waste products from the blood by filtering them into the urine.

Lipids: Complex fats used in the body to store and transport needed minerals.

Metabolic rate: The rate at which the body performs its chemical and physical functions.

Metabolism: All of the chemical and physical changes in the body that enable it to grow and function.

Minerals: Substances needed in small amounts to build and repair body tissues and/or to control functions of the body. Calcium, iron, potassium, and magnesium are examples of minerals.

Monounsaturated fat: Fat that tends to lower blood cholesterol. Olive oil and canola oil are good sources of monounsaturated fats.

Nephropathy: Kidney disease. People who have had diabetes for many years are at risk of getting nephropathy.

Neuropathy: Nerve disease. Often causes loss of sensation or movement and pain or burning in the feet and legs. May also affect nerves in other parts of the body. People who have had diabetes for many years and/or poor blood glucose control are at risk of getting neuropathy.

Nutrient: A substance in food that is needed by the body. Proteins, fats, carbohydrates, minerals, vitamins, and water are examples of nutrients.

Ophthalmologist: A medical doctor who specializes in the care and treatment of eye diseases.

Optometrist: A specialist who is trained to examine the eyes and prescribe lenses or exercises to correct vision problems.

Pancreas: An organ that produces insulin, digestive enzymes, and other hormones.

Polydipsia: Increased thirst. A symptom of hyperglycemia.

Polyunsaturated fat: Fat that tends to lower blood cholesterol. Found in most vegetable oils. Soybean oil, cottonseed oil, corn oil, and peanut oil are all good sources of polyunsaturated fats.

Polyphagia: Increased appetite. A symptom of hyperglycemia. Can also accompany hypoglycemia.

Polyuria: Increased urination. A symptom of hyperglycemia.

Protein: A nutrient found in food. Proteins are building blocks and a source of energy.

Psychologist: A health care professional who has specialized training in the treatment of problems that cause mental and emotional distress.

Retinopathy: A disease of the retina in the eye. A complication of diabetes.

Saturated fat: Fat that tends to raise the cholesterol level in the blood. Usually found in foods that come from animals. Butter and lard are saturated fats. Some vegetable oils, such as palm oil and coconut oil, are also saturated fats.

Signs: An abnormal finding, such as fever based on a temperature reading.

Social worker: A person with specialized training in helping individuals and families to solve practical and emotional problems.

Symptoms: An abnormal sensation or physical complaint, such as abdominal pain.

Type 1 diabetes: An autoimmune disease where the pancreas makes insufficient insulin.

Type 2 diabetes: A disease where the body is unable to use insulin properly.

Vitamins: Substances needed in small amounts for normal body growth and functioning.

Resources

Some of the resources listed below are for all people with diabetes, not just children. They are included here because you may have another family member with diabetes, or you may find them helpful later.

Some of the ADA books listed after the Index are particularly helpful for children with diabetes.

Other books by Jean Betschart Roemer that you might also find helpful:

> *It's Time to Learn About Diabetes* (Wiley & Sons)
> *In Control: A Guide for Teens* (Wiley & Sons)
> *Diabetes Care for Babies, Toddlers, and Preschoolers: A Reassuring Guide* (Wiley & Sons)
> *Type 2 Diabetes in Teens: Secrets for Success* (Wiley & Sons)

For General Questions

American Diabetes Association
1701 North Beauregard Street
Alexandria, VA 22311
800–Diabetes (800–342–2383)
703–549–1500
www.diabetes.org
A large repository of information about diabetes and living with diabetes

Children With Diabetes
www.childrenwithdiabetes.com
An online community for kids, families, and adults with diabetes

Joslin Diabetes Center
One Joslin Place
Boston, MA 02215
617–732–2400
800–567–5461
www.joslin.org
Detailed information about all types of diabetes

Juvenile Diabetes Research Foundation
26 Broadway
New York, NY 10004
800–533–2873
212–785–9595 (fax)
www.jdrf.org
Detailed information about type 1 diabetes

National Institute of Diabetes and Digestive and Kidney Diseases
Building 31, Room 9A06
31 Center Drive, MSC 2560
Bethesda, MD 20892–2560
301–496–3583
http://www2.niddk.nih.gov
Information about diabetes and related diseases

For Finding Quality Health Care

American Association for Marriage and Family Therapy
112 South Alfred Street
Alexandria, VA 22314
703–838–9808
703–838–9805 (fax)
www.aamft.org
For marriage and family therapists in your area go to:
www.therapistlocator.net/

American Association of Diabetes Educators
200 West Madison Street, Suite 800
Chicago, IL 60606
312–424–2426
312–424–2427(fax)
800–338–3633
www.diabeteseducator.org
To find local diabetes educators, go to: www.diabeteseducator.org/
DiabetesEducation/Find.html

American Association of Sex Educators, Counselors, and Therapists
P.O. Box 1960
Ashland, Virginia 23005–1960
804–752–0026
804–752–0056 (fax)
www.aasect.org
For a list of certified sex therapists and counselors in your state, go to:
www.aasect.org/directory.asp

American Board of Medical Specialties
222 North LaSalle Street, Suite 1500
Chicago, IL 60601
312–436–2600
http://www.abms.org
Record of physicians certified by 24 medical specialty boards. Check
online at www.abms.org/wc/login.aspx, or call the toll–free ABMS
Certification Verification Service at 1–866–ASK–ABMS (275–2267.)
Only certification status of physician is available to callers.

American Board of Podiatric Surgery
445 Fillmore Street
San Francisco, CA 94117–3404
415–553–7800
www.abps.org
Referral to a local board–certified podiatrist. To find a doctor, go to:
www.abps.org/content/resources/FindADoctor.aspx

American Dietetic Association
120 South Riverside Plaza, Suite 2000
Chicago, IL 60606–6995
800–877–1600
312–899–0040
www.eatright.org
Information, guidance, and referral to a local dietitian

American Medical Association
515 N. State Street
Chicago, IL 60654
800–621–8335
http://www.ama–assn.org
To find a physician, go to:
http://extapps.ama–assn.org//doctorfinder/recaptcha.jsp

American Optometric Association
243 N. Lindbergh Boulevard
St. Louis, MO 63141
314–991–4100
314–991–4101 (fax)
800–365–2219
www.aoa.org
To find an optometrist, go to: www.aoa.org/x5428.xml

American Psychiatric Association
1000 Wilson Boulevard, Suite 1825
Arlington, VA 22209–3901
703–907–7300
888–357–7924
www.psych.org
Referral to your state psychiatric association for referral to a local psychiatrist

American Psychological Association
750 First Street NE
Washington, DC 20002–4242
202–336–5500
800–374–2721
www.apa.org
Referral to your state psychological association for referral to a local
psychologist

National Association of Social Workers
750 First Street NE, Suite 700
Washington, DC 20002–4241
202–408–8600
http://www.naswdc.org
Referral to your state chapter of NASW for referral to a local social
worker

Pedorthic Footwear Association
2025 M Street, NW
Suite 800
Washington, DC 20036
202–367–1145
800–673–8447
Referral to a local certified pedorthist (a person trained in fitting
prescription footwear)

For Miscellaneous Health Information

American Academy of Ophthalmology
P.O. Box 7424
San Francisco, CA 94120–7424
415–561–8500
415–561–8533 (fax)
http://www.aao.org
For brochures on eye care and eye diseases, send a self–addressed,
stamped envelope

American Chronic Pain Association
P.O. Box 850
Rocklin, CA 95677
800–533–3231
916–632–3208 (fax)
http://www.theacpa.org
To learn more about chronic pain and how to deal with it

American Heart Association
7272 Greenville Avenue
Dallas, TX 75231
800–242–8721
www.heart.org
For referral to local affiliate's Heartline, which provides information on cardiovascular health and disease prevention

Medic Alert Foundation
2323 Colorado Avenue
Turlock, CA 95382
888–633–4298
www.medicalert.org
To order a medical ID bracelet

National AIDS Hot Line
Centers for Disease Control and Prevention
800–342–2437 (24 hours)
800–344–7432 (Spanish)
http://www.cdc.gov/hiv/
Information on HIV and AIDS, including pamphlets and brochures, counseling, and referral to local test sites, case managers, and medical services

National Kidney Foundation
30 E. 33rd Street
New York, NY 10016
212–889–2210
212–689–9261 (fax)
800–622–9010
www.kidnet.org
For donor cards and information about kidney disease and transplants

United Network for Organ Sharing
700 North 4th Street
Richmond, VA 23219
804–782–4800
804–782–4817 (fax)
888–894–6361
For information about organ transplants and a list of organ transplant
centers in the U.S.

For Travelers

American Diabetes Association
1701 North Beauregard Street
Alexandria, VA 22311
800–Diabetes (800–342–2383)
www.diabetes.org/living–with–diabetes/complications/frequent–
travelers.html
Up–to–date information to help travelers with diabetes

International Association for Medical Assistance to Travelers
1623 Military Road, #279
Niagara Falls, NY 14304–1745
716–754–4883
http://www.iamat.org
For a list of doctors in foreign countries who speak English and who
received postgraduate training in North America or Great Britain

International Diabetes Federation
Chaussée de la Hulpe 166
B–1170 Brussels, Belgium
+32–2–5385511
+32–2–5385114 (fax)
www.idf.org
For a list of International Diabetes Federation groups that can offer
assistance when you're traveling

For Exercisers

American College of Sports Medicine
P.O. Box 1440
Indianapolis, IN 46206–1440
317–637–9200
317–634–7817 (fax)
www.acsm.org
For information about health and fitness

Diabetes Exercise and Sports Association
310 West Liberty, Suite 604
Louisville, KY 40202
502–581–0207
502–581–0206 (fax)
http://www.diabetes–exercise.org
For people with diabetes and for health care professionals interested in
exercise and fitness at all levels

President's Council on Physical Fitness, Sports, and Nutrition
1101 Wooton Parkway
Suite 560
Rockville, MD 20852
240–276–9567
240–276–9860 (fax)
http://www.fitness.gov
For information about physical activity, exercise, and fitness

For Equal Employment Information

American Bar Association
Commission on Mental and Physical Disability Law
740 15th Street NW
Washington, DC 20005–1009
202–662–1570
202–442–3439 (fax)
800–285–2221
www.abanet.org/disability
Provides information and technical assistance on all aspects of
disability law.

American Diabetes Association
1701 North Beauregard Street
Alexandria, VA 22311
800–Diabetes (800–342–2383)
www.diabetes.org/advocate/
A large repository of patient advocacy information for people
with diabetes

Disability Rights Education and Defense Fund
2212 6th Street
Berkeley, CA 94710
510–644–2555
510–841–8645 (fax)
800–348–4232
http://www.dredf.org
Provides technical assistance and information to employers and
individuals with disabilities on disability rights legislation and policies.

Equal Employment Opportunity Commission
131 M Street, NE
Washington, DC 20507
800–669–4000
www.eeoc.gov

National Dissemination Center for Children With Disabilities
1825 Connecticut Avenue, NW
Suite 700
Washington, DC 20009
202–884–8200
202–884–8441 (fax)
800–695–0285
www.nichcy.org
Provides technical assistance and information on disabilities and
disability–related issues

For Health Insurance Information

American Diabetes Association
1701 North Beauregard Street
Alexandria, VA 22311
800–Diabetes (800–342–2383)
www.diabetes.org/living–with–diabetes/treatment–and–care/health–
insurance–options
Information from ADA about insurance options

Centers for Medicare and Medicaid Services
7500 Security Boulevard
Baltimore, MD 21244–1850
800–633–4227
www.medicare.gov
For information and various publications about Medicare

American Diabetes Association—National Office
1701 North Beauregard Street
Alexandria, VA 22311
800–Diabetes (800–342–2383)
(703) 549–1500
www.diabetes.org

ADA Regional Offices

Alabama
Birmingham   205–870–5172

Alaska
Anchorage   907–272–1424

Arizona
Phoenix   602–861–4731
Tucson   520–795–3711

Arkansas
Bentonville   479–464–4121
Little Rock   501–221–7444

California
Costa Mesa   714–662–7940
Los Angeles   323–966–2890
North Highlands 916–924–3232
Oakland   510–654–4499
San Diego   619–234–9897
San Jose   408–241–1922

Colorado
Denver   720–855–1102

Connecticut
Rocky Hill   203–639–0385

Delaware
Wilmington   302–656–0030

District of Columbia
Washington DC 202–331–8303

Florida
Fort Lauderdale 954–772–8040
Jacksonville   904–730–7200
Maitland   407–660–1926
Miami   305–477–899
Pensacola   850–492–6100
Tampa   813–885–5007

Georgia
Atlanta   404–320–7100
Savannah   912–353–8110'

Hawaii
Honolulu   808–947–5979

Illinois
Chicago   312–346–1805
Springfield   217–875–9011

Indiana
Evansville   812–476–6949
Indianapolis   317–352–9226

Iowa
Cedar Rapids   319–247–5124
Urbandale   515–276–2237

Kentucky
Lexington   800–676–4065 x3327
Louisville   502–452–6072

Kansas
Overland Park 913–383–8210
Wichita   316-684–6091
Louisiana
Baton Rouge 225–216–3980
Metairie   504–889–0278

Maine
Portland   207–774–7717

Maryland
Baltimore   410–265–0075

Massachusetts
Boston   617–482–4580

Michigan
Bingham Farms 248–433–3830
Grand Rapids   616–458–9341

Minnesota
St. Louis Park 763–593–5333

Mississippi
Jackson   601–366–1763

Missouri
St. Louis   314–822–5490
Springfield   417–890–8400

Montana
Billing   406–256–0616

Nebraska
Omaha   402–571–1101

Nevada
Henderson   702–369–9995

New Jersey
Bridgewater   732–469–7979

New Mexico
Albuquerque 505–266–5716

New York
Albany   518–218–1755
Amherst   716–835–0274
East Syracuse 315–438–8687
Melville   631–348–0422
New York   212–725–4925
Rochester   585–458–3040
Utica   315–735–6434
White Plains   914–253–4909

North Carolina
Charlotte   704–373–9111
Raleigh   919–743–5400

North Dakota
Fargo   701–234–0123

Ohio
Akron   330–835–3149
Cincinnati   513–759–9330
Columbus   614–436–1917
Independence 216–328–9989

Oklahoma
Oklahoma City 405–840–3881
Tulsa   918–492–3839

Oregon
Eugene   541–343–0735
Portland   503–736–2770

Pennsylvania
Bala Cynwyd 610–828–5003
Bethlehem   610–814–2701
Harrisburg   717–657–4310
Pittsburgh   412–824–1181

Rhode Island
Providence   401–351–0498

South Carolina
Columbia   803–799–4246
Greenville   864–609–5054

Tennessee
Knoxville   865–524–7868
Memphis   901–682–8232
Nashville   615–298–3066

Texas
Austin   512–472–9838
Corpus Christi 361–850–8778
Dallas   972–255–6900
Edinburg   956–631–1118
Houston   713–977–7706
Lubbock   806–794–0691
Midland   432–570–1232
San Antonio   210–829–1765

Utah
Salt Lake City 801–363–3024

Virginia
Chesapeake   757–424–6662
Glen Allen   804–225–8038

Washington
Richland   509–943–0858
Seattle   206–282–4616
Spokane   509–624–7478

Wisconsin
Brookfield   414–778–5500
Monona   608–222–7785

Index

Other Titles from the American Diabetes Association

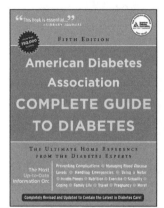

Complete Guide to Diabetes, 5th Edition
by American Diabetes Association

Have all the tips and information on diabetes that you need close at hand. The world's largest collection of diabetes self-care tips, techniques, and tricks for solving diabetes-related problems is back in its fifth edition, and it's bigger and better than ever before.

Order no. 4809-05; Price $22.95

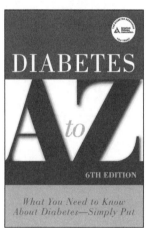

Diabetes A to Z, 6th Edition
by American Diabetes Association

If you want the ins and outs of diabetes without the confusing jargon, then *Diabetes A to Z* is your go-to resource. *Diabetes A to Z*, 6th Edition, contains the most up-to-date recommendations by the American Diabetes Association, presented in a simple, yet informative, format. Get your answers to all your questions quickly and get back to living your life.

Order no. 4801-06; Price $16.95

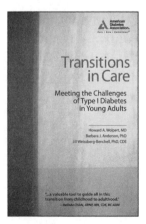

Transitions in Care
by Howard A Wolpert, MD; Barbara J. Anderson, PhD; and Jill Weissberg-Benchell, PhD, CDE

Transitioning from teenage years to adulthood is even tougher for young adults with type 1 diabetes. *Transitions in Care* serves as a coaching manual and self-care guide to help make the passage to adulthood easier for everyone involved.

Order no. 5438-01; Price $24.95

Lickety-Split Diabetic Meals *by Zonya Foco, RD, CHFI, CSP*

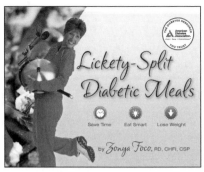

Let Zonya Foco be your guide as you learn how to save time, eat smart, lose weight, and win the war against obesity, diabetes, and heart disease. You'll get over 175 recipes and meals that can be prepared in minutes. *Lickety-Split Diabetic Meals* is a one-of-a-kind resource for people with diabetes and can help you learn how to change the life you have into the life you want.

Order no. 4669-01; Price $18.95

What Do I Eat Now?

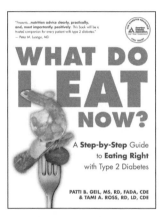

by Patti B. Geil, MS, RD, FADA, CDE, and Tami A. Ross, RD, LD, CDE
You've been told to eat healthy, but what does that mean? With this book, you'll know exactly what it means. In only 4 weeks, you will learn how to eat better, improve diabetes management, and live a healthier lifestyle.
Order no. 4886-01; Price $17.95

487 Really Cool Tips for Kids with Diabetes

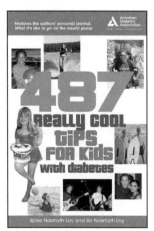

by Spike Nasmyth Loy and Bo Nasmyth Loy
This book is packed full of practical, real-world tips that kids, parents, and doctors around the world have sent to the two authors of *Getting a Grip on Diabetes*. Helpful tips cover everything from playing sports to accidents to hormones. Plus, there's an entire section on insulin pumps.
Order no. 4913-01; Price $14.95

To order these and other great American Diabetes Association titles, call 1-800-232-6733 or visit http://store.diabetes.org. American Diabetes Association titles are also available in bookstores nationwide.